From Fatty Liver to Healthy Liver

I Reversed My Fatty Liver Naturally. Learn How to Do It Too!

by

Lynn Luciano

www.FattyLiverDiary.com

Disclaimer and terms of use

This book is for informational and educational purposes only. It was not written by a medical practitioner: the author was diagnosed with a fatty liver disease and reversed it. The information in this book should not be considered a substitute for professional medical advice.

Always consult with your physician or another qualified healthcare provider before attempting to change your diet, take supplements, or begin an exercise program, and never stop or change any prescription medications or any other type of treatment without consulting your physician or qualified healthcare provider first.

This book is independently authored and the author assumes no responsibility or liability whatsoever on behalf of any reader of this book. Any use of the information in this book is made on the reader's good judgment and is their own sole responsibility. This book is not intended to treat any condition (or diagnose it), and should not be considered a substitute for a physician's advice or opinion. Individual results may also vary.

All attempts have been made by the author to provide factual and accurate information, based on personal experience reversing the disease, as well as in-depth research spanning over several years. However, the author does not assume any responsibility for errors of any kind, unintentional mistakes, or interpretations of the subject matter. Your purchase of this book and its use thereof means that you acknowledge and agree with everything mentioned above and you hold the author harmless for any potential consequences of your actions taken based on the information you find in this book. The purchaser and/or reader of this book assumes complete responsibility for the use of materials and information found in this book.

Dedication

This book is dedicated to my wife, Alina, and my son, Eric. Thank you for all the support you offered during and after my journey to reverse my fatty liver disease!

Table of Contents

1.Introduction

My name is Calin, though people call me Lynn because it's easier. Like many of you, I was diagnosed with a fatty liver disease. When my doctor delivered the news, she said my best hope was to keep the disease under control and prevent it from worsening. She told me it couldn't be healed or reversed. Today, however, I am here to tell you that you actually CAN reverse your fatty liver!

I did it!

As the title of the book suggests, I managed to reverse my non-alcoholic fatty liver disease - NAFLD, now called MASLD (metabolic dysfunction-associated steatotic liver disease) - in about 18 months. It might have happened sooner, but that's when I got confirmation from my hepatologist that my liver had indeed returned to normal and all my test results were good.

I decided to write this book with one main goal: to help you reverse your fatty liver too. Everything in this book is based on my personal experience with the disease, through direct experience, research, and discussions with other patients and experts. I detail all the steps I took to reverse my condition and offer advice on what you can do to reverse yours.

Since my diagnosis in 2014, I have continuously learned about fatty liver and helped others reverse their conditions. Many who have followed my advice have successfully reversed their conditions, according to their posts in the Facebook liver support group I manage (Reverse Fatty Liver: Support Group) and on my personal blog (Fatty Liver Diary - be sure to check it out!). Hopefully, now that this book is a reality, even more people will benefit from my knowledge.

The sad truth is that diagnoses of fatty liver disease have become more and more common these days, for patients of all ages. However, the fact that this problem is so common doesn't mean it should be ignored are taken lightly, as some doctors unfortunately do. On the contrary, it highlights that we humans are becoming sicker and unhealthier, and this needs to change!

Fortunately, you are taking direct action by choosing to read this book. This is one of the most important steps toward curing yourself - being proactive - so congratulations for doing this!

Of course, simply reading the book is not enough to get your health back on track, but it does set the foundation and helps you make the right choices to become healthy once more. It can also empower you to help others around you regain their health.

How will this book help you? It will provide all the information you need to make informed choices about reversing your fatty liver disease and becoming a healthier person overall. You'll learn what to eat, what to avoid, and how to stay motivated and healthy even after reversing your condition.

This book will guide you through all the steps needed to reverse your fatty liver and explain in easy-to-understand English why you should do certain things and not others. It will also offer various options and routes to take, so you can choose the one that best fits your situation.

The nice thing about MASLD (or fatty liver disease, or liver steatosis, or however you choose to call it) is that there isn't just one way to cure it: various approaches work, so you do have options.

Before we get into this, a quick note: I am not a native English speaker. This means my vocabulary and grammar may not be perfect, and there might be minor (or even major) mistakes despite my best efforts.

Even though the presentation might not be as charming and polished as I'd like, I strive to offer information that is correct and accurate. The core message should not be affected by my potential inability to write as well as a native speaker. I hope you can understand and accept this minor issue - and for that, I thank you! I am sure you won't regret it.

That being said, it's time to start working on improving your health and reversing your fatty liver. It might sound cliché, but it's true: If I did it, you can do it too! All you need is the correct information and the right amount of motivation to achieve your goal, and that's what I plan to deliver based on all my personal experience and research.

1.1 My Fatty Liver Story

I was diagnosed with a fatty liver back in September 2014 during a routine checkup. I wasn't expecting it, although I had been feeling unwell for a while before deciding to visit my doctor. What followed was an emotional whirlwind that almost crushed me - probably very similar to how you felt when you were first diagnosed.

I still vividly remember the horrible, terrifying feelings I had when the hepatologist started telling me during the ultrasound that my liver was enlarged. There was fat in my liver, fat in my pancreas, and fat around my kidneys.

"Things are not looking good," she said. That's when I felt the entire weight of the world on my shoulders.

I was scared. I was mortified, actually. I didn't know what all those things meant, but it didn't sound good. Having my father succumb to a liver-related illness just a few years before made things even worse.

The doctor told me that I had a fatty liver and that further tests were needed to determine how bad it was. She looked at me and told me there was nothing I could do to fix this and my best hope was for it not to progress into something worse. My heart sank.

She started talking about diets that I had to follow, recommending things to eat, things to avoid, and lifestyle changes I should make. But everything happened so fast, so quickly after the initial scare, that I didn't understand much. By the time I left her office, I had already forgotten most of what she told me.

All I understood, still in shock, was this: I was going to die. I couldn't think about anything else. I knew nothing about fatty liver, what it meant, or how serious of a disease it was. I already had a doctor telling me there was nothing I could do about it.

I remember getting back home, in a daze, depressed and scared. I burst into tears. I was crying my heart out. I was afraid I was going to lose everything. I was afraid I would miss out on so much: seeing my newborn son grow into an amazing man and being around to help him achieve this, growing old next to my beautiful wife and enjoying life with her, developing into a better person, and so much more.

I was about to turn 30. It was too early!

But even though the doctor herself told me there was nothing to do to heal my liver, and even though I thought she meant it was game over for me sooner rather than later, I decided to start doing my own research and see if there might be hope. I'm not one to go down without a fight. I'm not one to just quit without giving it my best, especially when I have so much to lose!

It didn't take a lot of research to start getting my hopes up. There were many doctors, patients, studies, and random people out there claiming that fatty liver can be reversed. That you can heal your liver completely. That you can get past this and get your life back. So I read more and more.

Hope!

I now had a single goal in life: to get healed. For my son. For my family. For myself.

And so I did.

Eighteen months later, after changing my pessimistic (and most likely not-so-well-trained) hepatologist with an amazing one who kept encouraging me and congratulating me on my progress, I got the news that I had indeed reversed my fatty liver.

After just eighteen months, I managed to turn this nightmare into one of the best things that ever happened to me. I had gotten my life back. I had reversed my fatty liver and gained a lot more than that: I was feeling better than ever, full of energy, happy, and well. I was healthy. I was ecstatic.

My doctor was happy too. "You should tell everybody about this," she said jokingly. "You should share your story with all my patients so they know they can do this."

So I decided to follow her advice. Over the years, even before launching this book, I helped others with advice that led them to reverse their fatty liver or at least improve their condition. Now I want to do it on a larger scale with the help of this book.

Even if there's just one person reading this book who feels the way I did when I was diagnosed, and I can help them heal their liver, get healthy, and regain their life, then I am extremely happy.

Because that person - YOU - can share the knowledge with another, then another, and together we can heal the world, "pay it forward" style.

Let's start with YOU now!

2. Understanding Fatty Liver

In some cases, even doctors have a hard time pinpointing the specific cause of fatty liver disease. They usually blame genetics when the cause isn't clear, but in most cases, it's relatively simple for them to guess why you developed it.

Usually, a non-alcoholic fatty liver - since this is what this book is about - is caused by poor eating and lifestyle choices.

I was well overweight when I was diagnosed and living a chaotic life: eating processed foods high in fats and sugars, drinking alcohol regularly (although moderately), especially when going out with friends, getting no exercise, and lacking sleep. Without knowing, I was destroying my body. And I am sure I'm not the only one in that situation.

For others, fatty liver is caused by other existing conditions, from diabetes and other health problems to various pills and medications used to treat them.

But most of the time it's us being overweight, inactive,

stressed, eating mostly unhealthy foods, and drinking alcohol.

The easiest way to defeat an illness is to first understand it and then deal with what's causing it. I won't go too in-depth with this section - the purpose of this book is to help you reverse fatty liver, not go through all the medical details and specifics of the condition. Also, you probably know what it is already and the reversing it part is more important.

But still, we should go through some basics first, as they will help you make correct choices later.

2.1 What Is Fatty Liver Disease / MASLD?

Non-alcoholic fatty liver disease, also known as fatty liver disease NAFLD or MASLD, is the term used for an excessive buildup of fat in the liver. This problem is becoming increasingly common: it is estimated that up to 30% of the American population suffers from a form of fatty liver (up from 20% when I was diagnosed - a 10% increase in around 10 years!). In fact, it is the most common form of chronic liver disease in the developed world.

However, since there are usually no signs or symptoms, exact numbers can't be known as many might have it without being aware. One thing is clear: more and more people suffer from fatty liver as our lives become more sedentary and our diets increasingly consist of highly processed and unhealthy foods.

There are two types of fatty liver disease:

- **Non-alcoholic fatty liver disease (NAFLD):** This is the most common type and occurs when the buildup of fat in the liver is not directly related to alcohol consumption.

- **Alcoholic fatty liver disease (AFLD):** This type affects heavy drinkers. As a result of excessive alcohol consumption, the liver gets damaged and can no longer break down fats as it's supposed to, resulting in a buildup of fat in the liver.

When too much fat is stored in liver cells, it can cause inflammation and damage, leading to scarring (fibrosis) which can progress to cirrhosis or liver failure if not addressed.

The condition was initially known as NAFLD (non-alcoholic fatty liver disease) but has been reclassified to MASLD to emphasize its association with metabolic dysfunction, including obesity, type 2 diabetes, hyperlipidemia (high levels of fat in the blood), and hypertension.

This reclassification also highlights that the disease can affect individuals who are not obese, focusing attention on the broader metabolic factors involved.

Even though fatty liver, especially in its early stages, is not a life-threatening problem, it can potentially become one, so it's best to address it as quickly as possible. Also, many patients may suffer from fatty liver for several years without it developing into something more serious. However, you can never know for sure how your body will react to it, so it's best not to risk it.

Many doctors downplay the importance of fatty liver because of this, and as a result, many patients fail to reverse it, especially since major lifestyle changes are required. For example, I wouldn't have reversed my condition if I had only listened to the first hepatologist I visited, who told me that it's a condition that can't be cured.

We all need to understand that MASLD is a potentially life-threatening problem that must be addressed and reversed as soon as possible. It won't always be easy (although in some cases, it could be easier and faster than in mine), but starting NOW is essential. Ignoring it and allowing it to worsen for six months, a year, or longer will only make it more difficult to cure/reverse.

2.2 What Causes a Fatty Liver?

In the case of alcoholic fatty liver, excessive alcohol consumption is the primary culprit. Alcohol damages the liver, impairing its ability to process fat normally, which results in a buildup of fat within the liver.

In the case of a non-alcoholic fatty liver, it's not always easy to pinpoint the exact causes - as we have already discussed.

Usually, the primary reason people are diagnosed with fatty liver disease is obesity, which is a result of a sedentary lifestyle, overeating, and consuming unhealthy foods that are high in saturated fats, sugars, and artificial additives. All of these factors, over time, take their toll on our livers.

However, there are various other reasons why people might develop a fatty liver. Sometimes, genetics play a role, making individuals more susceptible.

Consuming foods that are high in fats and carbohydrates and are heavily processed - with added chemicals for improved taste, more appealing colors, and longer shelf life - can also lead to a fatty liver, even in people who are not overweight.

Conditions like diabetes, high levels of fats in the blood, and certain medications can cause MASLD or contribute to an excessive buildup of fat in your liver.

While it's uncommon, even thin, apparently healthy individuals can be diagnosed with a fatty liver. However, it is usually those who are obese, don't exercise, and consume unhealthy foods who are most at risk of developing this condition.

2.3 What Are the Symptoms of Fatty Liver?

In many cases, a fatty liver causes no symptoms, especially early on. Even blood tests can come back normal.

This was the case for me: my blood test results were normal (though many were close to the upper limit). Despite this, I was diagnosed with a fatty liver: my symptoms were the warning sign, and then the ultrasound confirmed the worries, which were later confirmed by a FibroScan.

Eventually, if you have a fatty liver, you will most likely experience one or more of the following symptoms:

- Pain in the upper right side of the abdomen, under the rib cage (this is one of the most common symptoms).
- Constant fatigue.
- Bloating.
- Nausea.
- Sweaty palms.
- Loss of appetite.
- Itchy skin (this can occur all over the body or in

specific areas, such as your back, belly, or hands).

- Red spots on the skin.

- Abdominal fullness and discomfort.

It is extremely important to consult a doctor if you experience any of these symptoms or if you believe you might have a fatty liver, even if no symptoms are present.

The symptoms listed above are pretty generic and may not always be the result of a fatty liver. Therefore, a physician with the proper medical expertise will know what tests to conduct to determine the cause of these symptoms. But never delay visiting the doctor! Better to be safe than sorry, as the earlier you detect a fatty liver (or most diseases, for that matter), the easier it is to treat.

Another important thing to have in mind is that the severity of the symptoms does not necessarily indicate that your condition is in a very advanced state or worsening.

In my case, a multitude of symptoms were present, some of which gradually worsened until I realized that something was indeed wrong and a visit to the doctor could no longer be delayed. Here's what I experienced:

1. Fatigue: This was my biggest problem early on. I always felt exhausted, tired, and grumpy. I was working many hours each day back then, so I initially thought that was the reason for my constant fatigue. It turned out not to be the case, especially since I now work the same hours and am nowhere near as tired as I was before being diagnosed and especially before reversing the condition.

2. Upper right side pain: This pain was the reason I made my doctor's appointment. It was a dull pain that sometimes subsided without any apparent reason and sometimes intensified, usually after eating fatty foods. This is one of the most common symptoms among people with fatty liver. The severity of the pain can vary greatly; some even report it being so severe that it wakes them up if they're sleeping. In my case, it was just a mild, annoying pain for most of the time, with more intense spurts every now and then.

The pain often persists even after starting to eat healthy and making the required lifestyle changes, but improves over time as the liver heals.

Some doctors usually say that the liver doesn't hurt and that the pain can't be caused by a fatty liver. However, many of the people I have spoken to who were suffering from MASLD said that they experienced pain in the upper right side as well - it can now be considered one of the most obvious symptoms of a fatty liver.

There might be a logical explanation for it. And that's fortunately not the fact that many doctors don't know what they're saying. What is causing the pain, generally, is the enlarged liver which starts pushing and pressing on other organs around it. Therefore, it causes pain, and even though it's not the liver itself that hurts, it is the reason why you feel this pain in the first place.

3. Bloating: I was always bloated, which I attributed to my lifestyle. I was eating extremely unbalanced and unhealthy meals,

I was drinking soda constantly and I was overweight. I thought that was the reason why I was always bloated, but apparently, that might not have been the case.

4. Nausea: This symptom appeared later, with the first three symptoms having been present for a while before my visit to the hepatologist. Eventually, I started feeling nauseous after most meals, especially after eating large portions or very greasy/heavy foods. I had never experienced such issues before, which raised an alarm in my mind.

5. Your body sending alarm signals: Finally - I am not sure if I can consider this a symptom or not (or just me being crazy), but I started to feel the need to eat healthy food. I found myself craving soups (which I didn't normally eat) and fruits and vegetables (which I also didn't regularly consume).

So maybe those who advise us to listen to our bodies might know what they're sending. Our bodies may indeed send us signals when needed. However, it is crucial to consult a specialist and not rely solely on your body's messages - especially since most of us aren't trained to understand what these signals mean.

Back to the symptoms, although the consensus is that fatty liver disease can have no symptoms at all, most of the people I met who were diagnosed with it experienced a variety of the ones above, with pain under the right rib being the most common but usually not the only one.

Like many others before being diagnosed, they did not think these symptoms were related to anything specific, particularly as the symptoms tended to appear and disappear randomly. This is another reason to understand that whenever something doesn't feel right, you should schedule an appointment with your doctor!

2.4 How Is Fatty Liver Diagnosed?

Usually, fatty liver is diagnosed during routine checks if no symptoms are present. The easiest way to diagnose a fatty liver is by ultrasound, which can then be confirmed by a FibroScan. Other imaging studies, like CT or MRI scans, may be done, but typically, an ultrasound is sufficient to identify the condition.

A physical exam can also provide indications of a fatty liver. By simply examining your abdomen and pressing on the liver, a doctor can detect inflammation or an enlarged liver. However, confirmation still requires one of the imaging methods mentioned above.

Blood tests could also indicate the presence of a fatty liver, usually through increased liver enzymes (ALT and AST) and high cholesterol levels. However, further investigations are necessary to confirm or rule out the MASLD diagnosis.

As I mentioned earlier, you can have a fatty liver even if your blood test results are normal. If you have symptoms, multiple diagnostic methods will be used to ensure an accurate diagnosis.

After being diagnosed, most doctors will want to assess the severity of the fatty liver disease, which is typically categorized into three grades. In some cases, a liver biopsy may be requested. While it might sound scary, it involves the doctor inserting a needle into your liver to obtain a sample, with a local anesthetic used to minimize pain.

Alternatively, a less invasive method called FibroScan can be used. This was the method used in my case. FibroScan is a specialized, non-intrusive form of ultrasound imaging that can detect the severity of the condition without any pain and potential side effects.

2.5 Understanding the Three Stages of Fatty Liver Disease

Fatty liver disease can be classified into different stages or grades of severity, with lower numbers indicating less serious conditions. Grades 1 through 3 of fatty liver disease range from mild to severe, and the higher the number, the more time will be required to reverse it.

Grade 1 Fatty Liver: This is the mildest form of fatty liver disease but still indicates that your liver has an unhealthy amount of fat cells. Livers with five to thirty-three percent of fat cells contributing to the overall weight of the organ are considered to have grade 1 fatty liver disease.

In grade 1 fatty liver disease, the excess fat cells reside on the outside of the organ, accumulating in clusters on its surface. While unhealthy, the fat cells are not yet numerous enough to impact the function of the liver itself.

Most of the time, doctors can detect grade 1 fatty liver

disease with an ultrasound, and it's usually diagnosed during routine check-ups, as there might be no symptoms yet. Even blood test results can come back normal with grade 1 fatty liver, making it difficult to catch in most cases. However, if you do, it's also the easiest to reverse with the proper lifestyle changes.

Grade 2 Fatty Liver: This means that the fat cells in your liver make up thirty-four to sixty-six percent of your liver's weight. This condition is considered moderate and can progress from grade 1 fatty liver if left untreated.

Unlike grade 1 fatty liver, which doesn't affect the inner functioning of the liver, grade 2 fatty liver displays fat cells that begin to invade the liver cells and create ballooning pockets of fat. This slows down the liver's ability to metabolize nutrients from the stomach and intestines and get rid of toxins in the body.

Inflammation of the liver lobes may also begin to occur during grade 2 fatty liver disease. Additionally, blood test results might come back abnormal, and you might experience one or more symptoms associated with NAFLD.

This is the stage at which I was diagnosed, and I still managed to reverse my condition, so it's possible. It might take a bit longer to reverse from this stage, but still doable in as little as a few to several months.

Grade 3 Fatty Liver: This is considered the most severe stage of fatty liver before more serious problems might develop. When more than two-thirds of the liver's weight is comprised of fat cells, the diagnosis is grade 3 fatty liver disease.

Along with all the symptoms of grade 2 fatty liver disease, grade 3 is also marked by chronic inflammation of the liver. The difference between the inflammatory stages of grade 2 and grade 3 fatty liver is that grade 2 can involve episodic inflammation, while grade 3 inflammation is constant.

While there is no direct medication to treat fatty liver disease, all measures including lifestyle changes - especially switching to a healthy diet and exercising - are mandatory to get back in shape.

Left untreated for too long, a fatty liver in stage 3 can lead to much more serious health issues and permanent liver damage. Ultimately, it can become life-threatening, so it's not something to ignore.

However, grade 3 fatty liver can be reversed. It might not happen quickly - you will slowly regress to stage 2 and then stage 1 before full reversal. So start acting now to begin the healing process!

2.6 Can You Reverse Fatty Liver?

Fortunately, fatty liver disease is reversible, no matter what some people might tell you. The time it takes to reverse it can vary depending on how advanced it is and how committed you are to making the necessary lifestyle changes.

Staying motivated is the most important factor once you know what you need to do to reverse your fatty liver. So never lose momentum, never lose hope, and stick to it!

Remember that your journey to heal your liver is not a sprint, but a marathon. It usually requires a complete set of lifestyle changes - especially in your eating habits - and it's not going to be easy. But it is worth it!

For now, know this:

You can reverse your fatty liver disease! You can get healthy again. You can get your life back. Let's do it!

3. How to Reverse Fatty Liver

This is the most important part of the book. I didn't go too in-depth in the previous chapters because I believe that if you're reading this, you have already been diagnosed with a fatty liver and are more or less familiar with what it is. Plus, you're here to learn how to cure it, not to learn about it!

Now it's time to get serious and dive into the details. This is where most people get confused: how to reverse their fatty liver.

Everything you will read below is based on my own experience fighting against NAFLD/MASLD and eventually beating it, but also backed by hundreds of hours of research. The best part is that the methods I propose (which might be very similar to those recommended by good doctors or others who have successfully reversed their fatty liver) can be easily followed long-term. I say this because you should think long-term from now on. Even after reversing your condition, you have to keep eating healthy and staying active to ensure your liver remains healthy as well.

Reversing your fatty liver is just part of the challenge: an important one, it's true, but only part of it.

If you make all these changes to regain your health only to return to the old habits that caused the problem in the first place, the issues will return too. Fortunately, the methods I recommend and the lifestyle changes you need to make are not too strict and can become a sustainable, healthy way of living. I've been living by these principles since my diagnosis in 2014, and once you get used to the changes - it takes a few weeks - you won't want to get back to your old ways.

So, let's see how I managed to reverse fatty liver!

3.1 Develop the Right Mindset

Looking back at my situation in September 2014, when I was diagnosed, I realize that I had a terrible start: I returned home defeated, started crying, and was convinced I was going to die. For a very short time, I had given up all hope.

That's not how you do things! Negativity is not helpful. Negativity and a poor state of mind won't cure diseases. It's strong-willed people who succeed, so you have to develop the right mindset to make sure you'll do this!

I don't consider myself particularly strong-willed, and like many others, I've had my fair share of trouble with high stress and anxiety, all worsened by the constant feeling of being tired - a feeling caused by my sick liver. It wasn't an ideal situation, but hopefully, it proves that even if you don't consider yourself strong, you can still do it. We are always stronger than we think we are!

Right now, you might be in a situation similar to the one I was in when I was diagnosed, considering yourself too weak to do this, considering yourself already defeated. Right now, you might think that you don't have what it takes to be able to reverse your condition. It's too much, too hard. It requires too big of a change for you to be able to make it.

BUT THAT IS NOT TRUE. YOU ARE STRONG. YOU CAN DO IT!

This is the correct mindset. This is how you have to think. You need to tell yourself that you're strong. Because you are. I did it. Other people did it. It can be done. SO DO IT!

Even if you don't know it yet, you are a fighter. And you're not just any fighter: **you are a winner.** Winners are those who take action, and you've already taken the first and most important step by choosing to get this book and read it.

You can do it! I will help you do it. Your loved ones will help you. And even if you're all alone out there, you will still do it. Believe that, and say it to yourself every morning in the mirror until you feel it with every cell of your body. You. Can. Do. It.

Switching from my losing mindset, from my depression

after being diagnosed, to the correct mindset of a winner was not easy. But it happened after I had two major breakthroughs:

First, I read on the internet that you can reverse fatty liver disease. That was the first glimmer of hope, the spark that started the fire.

Second, I thought about my family. My son was 14 months old when I was diagnosed. I was almost 30 back then. I wanted to live. I had so many things to live for - just like everyone does. I wanted to see my son grow up. I wanted to grow old with my amazing wife. I wanted to travel the world, learn new things, experience new adventures, retire... everything people do nowadays.

There are so many things worth fighting for! Find the things that give you power. It doesn't matter if it's just one or if you have plenty of reasons to fight to regain your health. Find what matters to you and use it as fuel to keep going.

Even better, write those reasons down. Write them on a piece of paper and keep it within reach. Then read that piece of paper constantly. Whenever you're feeling down, whenever you start to think that dieting and exercising is too difficult, whenever you find yourself in a slump after eating something you shouldn't have - just go through your reasons once more, and motivation will return. Because even winners like yourself sometimes forget what the trophy they're fighting for actually is.

Remember: accepting defeat is not an option. Accepting defeat isn't even the easy way out, because it means more suffering for yourself and more suffering for the ones you love.

Never accept defeat, especially now, when dealing with your fatty liver! This is a problem that is so much easier to fix than many other challenges or illnesses.

Develop the right mindset, and you're already on the path to regaining your health. Do it for yourself! Do it for the ones you love! Do it for those who love you! Do it to give yourself extra chances to make all your dreams come true, to tick everything off your bucket list. And do it now!

3.2 How Long Does It Take to Reverse Your Fatty Liver?

While it took me 18 months to reverse my fatty liver, your journey might be quicker or take a bit longer, depending on the severity of your condition and other factors that you may or may not be able to influence.

I've spoken to people who have managed to fully heal their liver in just a few months. Some reversed their condition in several months, while others are still struggling years after being diagnosed.

On average, I would say that those who have successfully reversed their fatty liver needed around 12 months. However, some continue to struggle with the condition for years. These are often individuals who have difficulty sticking to their plans and diet. If you want to be a happy, successful story, you must understand and accept that there's no easy way out.

If you want to reverse your fatty liver disease, you have to work for it. The most important part is working on your diet. Trust me when I say that it's not as difficult as it seems, although it appears to be in your first few weeks.

Each person's life is different, and the healthier your lifestyle and eating habits are, the easier it will be for you to reverse your condition. However, since you've just been diagnosed with fatty liver (or have been fighting it for a while), chances are you don't currently live a healthy, active life. This will change. The new you will be completely different!

So, what to expect? Expect a challenging journey that will eventually become enjoyable. Expect a bumpy road ahead, a complete change in the things you eat, the way you live your life, and possibly even changes in your social circle and friendships (although these last two aren't a must).

Remember: You're doing this for yourself and your loved ones. Nothing else matters!

3.3 Foods to Stop Eating

In most cases, following a proper diet, eating healthy foods, and avoiding unhealthy choices are all you need to do to reverse your condition. There are a few types of food you must eliminate from your diet completely (unfortunately, the tasty, unhealthy ones), but I promise that you will end up loving healthy food and appreciating it more than you probably do now.

I want to start with the foods you should avoid because it's easier to remember them when planning your meals. Ideally, you should never touch them at all - but I know we're human, and every now and then, you might indulge. Just don't make it a habit! There are NO excuses to eat any of these foods more often than once in a blue moon.

As long as you avoid these foods like the plague, you can eat almost anything else in moderation. You will see that mixing and matching healthy foods becomes easier once you know exactly what you should stay away from... forever.

Here is the shortlist to make it easy to follow - I'll go in-depth and explain why each of these food types is on the list, but if you need to write them down somewhere, here is what you should write:

- Fried & deep-fried foods
- Foods with excessive fat, especially bad fats (red meats, cream, butter, etc.)
- Sugar and any food with added sugar (including fructose, dextrose, corn syrups, and other sugars)
- Juices (including freshly squeezed) and sodas (with added sugar)
- Highly processed foods
- Special mention: Grains (try to avoid them if you can't cut them out completely)
- Alcohol (not food, I know, but it has to be here!)

It might seem impossible to have a varied diet after reading this list, but you'll see that's not the case! It might also seem that you'll have to cut out everything that tastes good, but that's not true either. You'll realize this as you read this book, but for now, let's dive into the foods you should stop eating after being diagnosed with fatty liver disease (and learn why).

Fried or Deep-Fried Foods

I have a personal saying: if you have a fatty liver, don't even smell fried foods! That's how bad they are for your overall health, especially for NAFLD/MASLD.

From French fries to fried chicken, hamburgers, and even fried vegetables, anything cooked in oil, especially deep fried, and with a high-fat content (hence the presence of hamburgers on the list) should be eliminated from your diet.

I know this seems difficult. I loved fried foods, and the taste of your favorite dishes won't be the same when they're no longer fried - I can't sugarcoat this. But since it's your health on the line, this change is necessary.

It can be challenging, especially since many recipes begin with frying ingredients in oil, but it's possible to adapt. After I was diagnosed with a fatty liver, I went more than a year without eating any fried foods (not even sautéed), so it's perfectly doable, even if it's tough at first.

Now, my taste buds have adjusted, and I'm losing interest in fried foods altogether. In fact, I feel awful if I eat the greasy stuff I once loved. So yes, cooking without oil is possible, and food can still be delicious.

Why should you avoid deep-fried foods? The oil used for frying significantly increases the amount of fat - especially harmful saturated fat - in your food, along with the calories.

And what's one thing you don't need in excess right now? FAT! So cut this out of your diet, or you'll struggle to reverse the condition. Too much fat and too many calories don't align with healthy eating.

If you don't want to eliminate oil when cooking (as I did), you can use small amounts of healthy oils. Extra virgin olive oil should be your go-to oil from now on. Use less than any regular recipe calls for and less than what you're used to adding.

Just add enough to give a bit of flavor to your food, but never let the ingredients get soaked, and never deep fry them!

You'll lose some taste and crunchiness, but you'll gain in the health department.

For example, use a spray bottle to lightly coat your portion of vegetables if you really need to. (Truth: You don't!)

Never add more than a teaspoon of oil when cooking (for two portions, so a maximum of half a teaspoon per portion), and try cooking without any extra oil - you'll be surprised at how many foods still taste great without it!

Tip #1: Try roasting your vegetables or other foods in the oven instead of cooking them in a pan. They taste better when cooked without oil! Alternatively, consider getting an air fryer, which requires only tiny amounts of fat (if any) and still produces delicious meals.

Tip #2: If you need a base for cooking, replace oil with water to sauté vegetables, meat, and anything else. Just be sure to add extra water as it evaporates - a couple of tablespoons will disappear almost instantly from a pot on medium/high heat.

Tip #3: Spices! They are the secret weapon you have

against the new taste of your foods. Use plenty of healthy spices (make sure they are all-natural, not those mixes that are full of chemicals!) and you will find it easier to switch to fat-free cooking.

Foods with Added Sugars or High Carbohydrate Amounts

Sugar and foods that are high in carbohydrates are just as bad as plain fat. Some might even argue that foods with high-carb contents are worse than fat because they require extra processing in the liver, putting more pressure on the organ. And they still end up stored as fat.

All sweets you can buy in stores, restaurants, or anywhere else, as well as sugar itself, should be avoided or ideally eliminated from your diet. This includes all the alternative names for sugar or unhealthy sweeteners like dextrose, fructose, corn syrup, beet sugar, cane sugar, brown sugar, glucose, and so on, as well as foods with easily absorbed carbohydrates (like white bread).

Cakes, candies, and all foods with easily absorbed sugars should be eliminated or consumed only occasionally, and in small quantities. This includes homemade cakes and candy if they contain sugar, white flour, or other unhealthy ingredients (which they usually do!).

The American Heart Association recommends that, as of 2024, a healthy woman should consume no more than 6 teaspoons of added sugar (24 grams) per day, while a healthy man should limit intake to 9 teaspoons (36 grams) per day.

This might sound like a lot until you realize that a 12 oz Coca-Cola contains around 39 grams of sugar, while a single Snickers bar (1.56 oz or 44 grams) has 20 grams of sugar. As you can imagine, these will easily add up and have the potential to ruin any progress you've made.

I personally recommend striving to keep added sugar to a minimum - ideally, as close to 0 as possible. Remember: the numbers above are for healthy individuals, not those who already suffer from fatty liver disease. A fatty liver is already suffering, and processing extra sugar only makes things worse.

During my extreme dieting days, while I didn't count

carbs, I eliminated added sugar from my diet. I didn't buy anything with added sugar, and when cooking at home, I never added any sugar (except for a tiny bit of honey in my daily coffee until I was ready to drink it unsweetened).

I'm sure this was one of the key factors that helped me reverse my fatty liver. I did this for the first six months of dieting. Eventually, I started to allow myself bits of things with added sugars - but only bits, and even today I have multiple consecutive days when I eat nothing with added sugar or high-carb alternatives.

Apart from the few foods I buy or eat at restaurants where I have no control over the sugar content, I still never add sugar to anything I prepare myself (nor does my wife). I switched to using organic honey, but sparsely, as well as Stevia and more recently, erythritol or maltitol, which seems to be one of the best sugar alternatives available (more on this later).

Not eating sugar or the high fructose corn syrup and other sweeteners they're putting in everything nowadays is probably one of the most challenging parts of the fatty liver diet. You'll eventually get used to it but expect the first 2-3 weeks to be incredibly tough with intense cravings, especially if you have a sweet tooth like I do. It will be brutal, but it will get better!

Six months after eliminating sugar, I took a bite of a cake at my Grandmother's birthday party. It was my favorite cake, but I realized how insanely and unnecessarily sweet it was. So yes, even though it will be difficult, you'll adjust to not eating sugar, and you'll eventually realize just how excessive the sugar content is in foods you once considered normal.

IMPORTANT: You can still eat fruits because the human body is well-adapted to handling the sugar intake from fruits, as we've been eating these for millions of years. Fruits are not on the "easily absorbed sugars" list like regular sugars and sweeteners - but don't overdo it. Don't eat 5 pounds of bananas each day. Remember, moderation is key!

Also, don't consider natural fruit juices healthy or acceptable, even if you squeeze the fruits at home. When you do this, you strip away most of the fiber and many nutrients, leaving just the water and sugars in the fruit (the natural fructose), which become easily absorbed and as bad as raw sugar.

Don't add sugar to your coffee, and don't use sugars you think are healthier (like brown sugar) because they generally aren't, and the carbohydrate content is similar to that of regular sugar. Even the honey I use is mostly sugar, hence the reason why I only add it now and then in foods that truly need a sweet touch. So be very careful even with the healthier alternatives, and do your own research before switching to using these alternatives - check how many carbs there are per 100 grams (aim for a minimum of 60, ideally under 20).

Although extremely difficult, know this: if you can cut sugars off your diet, then the sky's the limit, and full health will soon follow! And even I don't like to say this, because you should always keep both under control, if you are to choose between something higher in fat vs higher in carbs, choose the former.

Highly Processed Foods

Processed foods, although convenient and often tasty, are detrimental to your overall health and especially harmful to your liver. These foods are typically high in fat or carbs, usually both. Usually, there's also a lot of salt too, which is never good in excess.

The list of "highly processed foods" is extensive and there are endless debates regarding this category, with some saying that almost everything we eat today or buy in stores is processed, like the fresh chicken breast we eat (because they're cut and packaged) or even ground coffee since it was processed in a factory.

Of course, we're not taking it to this extreme. If processed foods are made from natural ingredients only, without preservatives, added fats, or sugars, they might be safe to eat in moderation. Think about stuff like fruit bars (with zero sugar and just fruits and nuts) and anything else that might come in a bag, but it's all natural and healthy.

These healthier options are usually more expensive and may only be found in dedicated stores or sections of larger supermarkets, but they're worth considering for the sake of variety.

Most highly processed foods, including some that might seem healthy or at least neutral, like ready-made meals, white flour, white rice, snacks, crackers, cereals, sodas, and juices, should be avoided. The list is truly endless.

A good rule of thumb is this: if it comes in a bag, it's likely bad for you (this is a slight exaggeration, but it illustrates the point!). If there are 40 ingredients on the list and you need a degree in chemistry to understand one of them, it's bad for you. If the content of fat or sugar/carbohydrates is too high, it's bad for you. Preservatives, artificial flavorings, too much salt (sodium), and various additives are all bad for you.

So, always check the list of ingredients, or better yet, avoid these products altogether and learn to snack on healthier options like fruits, veggies, or nuts. It's difficult, I know, but it's the best approach.

Another reason to avoid highly processed foods is that they are often filled with chemicals, which can further damage your liver.

What does "too much" mean? It depends on your daily meal plan, but I generally avoid anything with more than 20 grams of fat and/or 20 grams of carbs per 100 grams when it comes to processed foods.

Remember, this rule applies specifically to highly processed foods. Fruits, for example, often have high carb values but are safe to eat in moderation. Nuts are also high in fats, but these are mostly healthy fats. So, this guideline is for processed foods only - and only for those that pass the first test of checking the list of ingredients.

However, always check the list of ingredients, and don't assume that something labeled or considered healthy is automatically safe for your liver. Two examples that come to mind are protein bars (which are often loaded with added sugars, though not always) and many gluten-free foods (which often replace gluten with sugars or other chemicals).

Foods High in Fat

Especially foods that are high in saturated fat. While many of these fall into the "highly processed foods" category, it's important to discuss them separately because many of the meats we commonly consume contain excessive, unhealthy amounts of fat.

Not all fatty foods should be treated equally, as we'll explore in the "What to Eat" chapter. There are so-called "healthy fats" (monounsaturated and polyunsaturated fats) that are essential for our well-being. What we need to avoid are foods high in saturated fat, such as butter, cheese, red meat (especially beef), bacon, lard, and cream.

The American Heart Association, for example, recommends a healthy person get no more than 5% to 6% of their daily calories from saturated fats. For a standard 2,000-calorie-per-day diet, this means that around 100-120 calories should come from saturated fats, which translates to around 13 grams of saturated fat to be consumed per day.

However, unlike added sugar, fat should not be eliminated from our diet. Healthy fats are vital for our bodies to function properly, and you can obtain these naturally from low-fat meats (like chicken breast or fish), avocados, nuts, and healthy oils (such as extra virgin olive oil), among other sources.

But remember that moderation is key here as well: polyunsaturated fats should account for no more than 10% of your daily calories, while monounsaturated fats should make up no more than 15%.

Grains

Grains fall into a gray area, so you'll see them mentioned both here and on the list of foods to eat. Not all grains are created equal. However, if you can eliminate most grains from your diet, you'd be doing yourself a favor. I know this is a difficult, maybe even impossible task since grains are a staple in most diets. I didn't eliminate all grains from my diet, but I did completely change the types of grains I consume.

What you should stop eating are highly processed cereal grains, such as white wheat, white rice, and even cornmeal. These grains have high carbohydrate contents and little nutritional value, and their production often involves the use of chemicals and bleaches that might cause more harm to a suffering liver.

Instead, switch to whole, less processed varieties, such as whole wheat flour, wild rice (brown, red, or black), rye, and oats, as well as foods from the pseudocereal category like chia seeds, amaranth, quinoa, and buckwheat.

3.4 Smoking and Drinking Alcohol

Smoking and drinking alcohol are delicate topics. In many cases, it's easier to stop eating fat or sugar than it is to quit smoking or drinking. However, if you want to get healthy, you must stop both. And I mean STOP, not just reduce the amounts consumed.

Even if your diagnosis is non-alcoholic fatty liver, as mine was, you still need to stop consuming alcohol - completely. Never touch it again. I know it seems difficult, even if you're just a social drinker, but it's necessary.

Some health experts and doctors may say that you might still be able drink some alcohol if you have a fatty liver, but what if they're wrong? What if that one glass of wine turns into cirrhosis ten years from now because you kept drinking "just" one glass of wine per week? Are you willing to take that risk? Hopefully not - I haven't, and I must say that even though I haven't touched alcohol since being diagnosed back in 2014, I still have a group of friends and a social life.

Why is alcohol bad for your liver?

When you consume alcohol, you put extra pressure on your liver to process it into acetic acid and then acetate, which can be safely eliminated from the body.

During this process, the liver can't focus on its main functions (like producing bile to help break down fats, storing and releasing glucose, and more). In the end, alcohol damages the liver and causes health problems - one of them being the buildup of fat in the liver.

Even a healthy liver has to work hard to break down alcohol and keep you safe, but a liver that's already suffering will suffer even more from the added stress and pressure. While it may seem logical that smaller quantities would have less impact than larger ones, you just don't want extra stress on your liver.

So there are two main reasons why you need to stop drinking alcohol if you have liver-related problems like NAFLD/MASLD:

1. **Additional liver stress:** When the liver breaks down

alcohol, the chemical reaction damages its cells, leading to inflammation and scarring.

2. **Bacterial invasion:** Alcohol damages the intestine, allowing bacteria from the gut to enter the liver. This bacteria, which shouldn't be there, causes even more damage to the liver.

These are just the direct effects. Indirectly, alcohol can also cause issues like high carbohydrate intake (especially from beer) and side effects such as losing self-control and eating large, unhealthy meals after drinking. Alcohol can quickly undo any progress you've made.

In other words, alcohol is unhealthy even for those who don't have fatty liver disease. Even the World Health Organization (WHO) recently updated its guidelines regarding alcohol consumption, concluding that "no level of alcohol consumption is safe for our health" even if you are an otherwise healthy individual.

While a healthy liver might handle some pressure if you

drink moderately, a liver that's already suffering can't. In this case, alcohol will at best delay the healing of your liver, but most likely will cause more damage. So please keep this in mind and don't risk your life on a glass of wine or beer or whatever type of alcohol you prefer!

This means that no alcohol is permitted if you have a fatty liver, even if your diagnosis is "non-alcoholic fatty liver."

You've probably heard about the health benefits of consuming moderate amounts of alcohol - this is often cited by those who still want to drink. But these claimed benefits aren't the whole story.

The supposed health benefits of moderate alcohol consumption (such as wine) generally apply only to healthy individuals.

Unfortunately, you're no longer in that category if you have a fatty liver. Your liver can't process alcohol as a healthy liver would, leading to a harmful spiral that worsens with each drink.

I recently read a study that compared the life expectancy of people who drink alcohol moderately to those who stop drinking entirely. The findings might seem surprising at first: those who stop drinking don't necessarily have an increased life expectancy; some actually have a shorter life expectancy than even moderate drinkers.

However, the key point is that people often stop drinking alcohol because they are forced to by health problems. If they had continued drinking, their lives would likely have been even shorter!

So, quitting alcohol helps them live longer, even if it doesn't mean living longer than healthy people who drink moderately/socially. This is crucial to understand - the whole story, not just the part that says "People who stop drinking live shorter lives than those who don't."

With this in mind, say no to alcohol. This includes all types, from low-alcohol beer to stronger spirits.

If you really need to replace alcohol with something - but

only AFTER you have reversed your fatty liver disease - you can occasionally have alcohol-free beer or wine (though the latter often contains plenty of other chemicals, so look for options without them if you can).

Remember that even without alcohol, these drinks are high in carbohydrates and calories, so it's still better to avoid them as much as possible. Also, make sure they have 0% alcohol, as some beers labeled as alcohol-free still contain a small amount of alcohol (usually under 1%, but still alcohol).

Can I at Least Drink Beer?

"Just a small bottle of beer. Can I drink that? Am I allowed to drink at least a glass of beer every now and then if I have a fatty liver? It can't do much damage, can it?"

These are common questions that arise after a period of dieting to reverse fatty liver. You don't have to be an alcoholic to miss the idea of drinking a cold beer on a hot summer's day.

Unfortunately, beer contains alcohol, so you will have to stop drinking it as well. Not even a beer, not even a glass. Not even a sip.

Could just a glass of beer do that much damage?

Of course, no one can say for sure how much actual damage drinking a single glass of beer per week, or per month or day, might do to your suffering liver. Due to its low alcohol content, it's possible that the damage wouldn't be significant.

But there are two important things to consider when looking at the big picture and planning for the future:

1. "Just a glass a month" can easily turn into "just one glass a week," then "just one more glass," and "one more now because it's a special occasion," until it eventually spirals out of control. This is too big of a risk!

The easiest way to approach this is simply to say no. It's similar to cookies or candy: it's much easier not to taste one than it is to stop after just one bite.

2. We don't know how much damage even a single glass of beer does to your liver. It could be minimal, but it could also be significant. Depending on the stage of your

fatty liver and how your body processes alcohol, the effects could be greater. Additionally, genetics might make you more susceptible to extra damage.

In the end, it comes down to this big question: **Are you willing to risk it?**

This is a question I encountered during my initial research after being diagnosed with a fatty liver. Someone was ready to take the risk - or so it seemed - but still needed validation from others. However, one response (that I'm recalling from memory) stood out:

"Are you willing to risk it all on a single glass of beer? It's your life that's at stake here. Maybe the effects won't be immediate. Maybe things won't get worse as soon as you finish your beer. But what if, 10 years from now, the damage done by it kills you? Are you ready to risk your life for a glass of beer?"

This was eye-opening for me and made me seriously reconsider my priorities and what truly matters in life. It kept me motivated and capable of avoiding alcohol since 2014, even after I reversed my fatty liver. Why risk it? That's the question I always ask myself whenever I'm tempted to consume something I shouldn't.

Giving up alcohol completely wasn't easy. But here I am, years later, having successfully reversed my fatty liver, feeling great and healthy, and still not drinking any type of alcohol. You should do the same if you care about your life.

Trust me when I say that avoiding alcohol won't ruin your social life as much as you might think. Most people will understand and accept your choices. And if your social life does take a hit because you stop consuming alcohol, that's actually a positive sign: it means you weren't hanging out with the right type of people anyway!

Yes, some friends might find it difficult to accept your new approach to life and your decision to say no to any type of drink. Even after all these years, I still have one friend who doesn't fully understand my choice and keeps trying to convince me that it's OK to have a beer every now and then. He's still a friend because we are really close, but those who couldn't understand have become acquaintances at best. Remember: it's all about priorities, and your own life should be far more important than maintaining toxic friendships.

Can You Drink Non-Alcoholic Beer?

While I've touched on this subject briefly, it's worth exploring in more detail because it's a nuanced situation. Opinions are divided on the safety of non-alcoholic beverages when you have MASLD, and ultimately, the choice is yours once you have all the information.

Personally, I didn't drink any type of alcohol or alcohol-free beverages until it was confirmed - 1.5 years after my diagnosis - that I had reversed my fatty liver disease. Afterward, I decided that I could occasionally treat myself to a non-alcoholic beer, usually on hot summer days or when I'm out with friends.

So far, it hasn't caused any apparent harm, but I limit myself to a maximum of three non-alcoholic beers in any given week, and I only have them on very rare occasions - definitely not weekly.

Overall, I recommend that anyone still working to reverse their condition avoid even non-alcoholic beers or wines until their fatty liver is reversed. These drinks still contain a lot of carbs and calories, which can make managing your caloric intake more challenging.

After you've reversed your fatty liver, resist the urge to start drinking alcohol again. If you really feel the need for something similar, try some of the non-alcoholic options available, but make sure they truly contain 0% alcohol. Some drinks labeled as alcohol-free can still have up to 0.5% alcohol.

This was my approach, and it seems to have worked well. It's your choice, but now you know what worked for me. And trust me - after months or years of not drinking alcoholic beverages, non-alcoholic ones will taste just like the real deal!

Also, be sure to check the list of ingredients. Many non-alcoholic drinks (especially wines, whiskeys, and other spirits) are actually blends of chemicals, which can be just as harmful as real alcohol. Stick to options made from natural ingredients only!

Smoking and Fatty Liver Disease

While we often think of cigarettes as primarily affecting the lungs, that's not entirely accurate, although the lungs do suffer the most. The smoke we inhale is filled with toxins, and the liver is responsible for removing most toxins from our bodies. As a result, many doctors believe that smoking adds extra stress and pressure on a fatty liver (or any liver, for that matter).

Although there are few medical studies specifically focused on the effects of smoking on a fatty liver, the consensus in the medical community is that even a few cigarettes per day can significantly harm a liver already compromised by disease. The same concerns apply to modern alternatives to cigarettes, like vaping.

One study I found, dating back to 2010, was conducted on rats. It showed that obese rats with fatty liver who were exposed to cigarette smoke (two cigarettes per day, five days per week, for four weeks) experienced an increase in the severity of their fatty liver.

Additionally, various medical sources claim that smoking is detrimental to a liver already suffering from a disease, including fatty liver disease.

My initial assumption - that the toxins from cigarette smoke pass through the liver, adding extra stress and causing further harm - seems to be supported by experts in the field.

But it's not just the toxins that are a concern. Cigarette smoke, particularly the nicotine in cigarettes, is also linked to high levels of fat in the blood. Smoking causes blood vessels to constrict, raising blood pressure and increasing the levels of fat in the body. This increases the risk of other health issues, such as high blood pressure, heart attack, or stroke.

If this doesn't seem directly related to the liver, consider this: the liver is responsible for producing cholesterol. A sick liver has an impaired ability to produce both good and bad cholesterol, which need to be balanced in the body.

Finally, while it's well known that smoking has

carcinogenic effects, I wasn't able to find specific studies linking smoking - or its carcinogenic effects - to the liver itself. However, it's always safer to assume the worst. Remember, since your liver is already compromised, it is more sensitive to harmful substances and behaviors than a healthy liver is.

Smoking also drains your energy, making it harder to keep up with exercise. Since adding exercise to your lifestyle is crucial after being diagnosed, cigarettes will only make it more challenging to get back in shape. So, just like with alcohol - you should stop smoking if you were diagnosed with a fatty liver disease.

3.5 The Fatty Liver Diet: What and How to Eat to Reverse Your Fatty Liver

Now that we've covered the basics, it's time to focus on what I consider the most important part of reversing fatty liver: the diet. In other words, what and how to eat to reverse your condition.

Since you already know what NOT to eat, this part should be a little easier: as long as you eat in moderation, anything that's not on the list of foods to avoid is allowed.

Yes, it might sound overly simple, but it's true. Of course, you can't just eat bananas, chicken breasts, or avocados all day - you need a balanced diet that includes a variety of foods to ensure you get all the nutrients your body needs.

Still, especially when you're just starting out and have so many things to consider (Does this food have too much fat? Too much sugar? Too many chemicals?), it can feel overwhelming.

While multiple approaches can work, I can only speak to

what I did and the diet I followed to reverse my condition. It's not a diet I created, but one I modified slightly to fully align with the guidelines of healthy eating for fatty liver while eliminating all the banned foods. It's also a diet that many other people diagnosed with fatty liver disease followed and reversed their condition. Let's take a look at it!

3.5.1 My (Slightly Modified) Mediterranean Diet

The Mediterranean Diet has been praised by countless health experts, doctors, and nutritionists as one of the healthiest diets in the world. Many experts consider it the best option for reversing fatty liver. This is the diet I decided to follow, making some minor adjustments to ensure you only get the good parts while avoiding the potentially harmful ones (like alcohol, for example).

My slightly modified approach to the Mediterranean Diet is the best choice you can make: it offers variety, tasty dishes, and a lot of options when it comes to what you can eat. So let's dive into it!

1. Fruits and Vegetables

These two categories should make up the majority of your diet, with vegetables being the bulk of your meals - whether it's breakfast, lunch, or dinner. Eat them raw, boiled, steamed, baked (without added fat), or grilled.

When it comes to vegetables, variety is key. However, you

still need to keep an eye on your carb intake, as some vegetables (often the tastiest ones) are high in carbohydrates. While you can still enjoy these higher-carb vegetables (because they also contain fiber, minerals, vitamins, and other nutrients), they shouldn't dominate your meals.

Here are some vegetables with the highest carbohydrate content per 100 grams. These should be consumed in smaller amounts during meals, but you can still enjoy them regularly:

- **Sweet Potatoes**: 23g

- **Potatoes**: 20g

- **Sweet Corn**: 19g

- **Parsnip**: 18g

- **Green Peas**: 14.5g

- **Acorn Squash**: 12g

Also, while not vegetables but often used as such, **plantains** have 32% carbs, and **cassava** (popular in some regions) has around 38 grams of carbs per 100 grams.

Most vegetables contain less than 10 grams of carbs per

100 grams, so they can be considered safe to eat. Even the higher-carb vegetables listed above are okay - especially when compared to raw sugar, which is 100% carbs, or regular chocolate, which can contain up to 60 grams of sugar per 100 grams.

As for fruits, you can still enjoy plenty because, although they have more carbs than vegetables, they also contain fiber and various other nutrients that benefit your health. As mentioned earlier, the fructose in fruits, combined with the other nutrients, is something our bodies have been processing for tens of thousands of years - so we're more accustomed to it than to processed sugars, which were introduced into our diets much later.

Like with vegetables, aim to consume more low-carb fruits than higher-carb ones. High-carb fruits include:

- **Bananas**
- **Grapes**
- **Melons**

- Mangoes

- Apples

- Pineapples

Lower-carb fruits include:

- **Watermelon**

- **Strawberries**

- **Cantaloupe**

- **Raspberries**

- **Oranges**

- **Peaches**

Since most fruits have under 20% carbs and are packed with fiber and other nutrients, they remain safe to eat in moderation. As I mentioned before, you shouldn't eat pounds of bananas each day and claim you're following a healthy diet! Instead, consume fruits as snacks between main meals (e.g., 1 banana, 1 apple, or a handful of berries), or add them in small amounts to yogurt, oatmeal, or porridge for the main meals of the day.

Also, eat whole fruits and vegetables. While smoothies are a good choice because they retain all the nutritional value of the ingredients, juices (even freshly squeezed at home) remove most of the fiber and nutrients, leaving mostly the sugar - so these should be avoided, if not completely eliminated, from your diet.

2. Legumes

Legumes are excellent as side dishes and can be a regular part of your meals too. They are high in protein and fiber, low in fats, and very filling, with lower carb values (usually under 15%, depending on the type).

Legumes to include in your diet, even in larger quantities, are all types of beans (such as red beans, cannellini, and kidney beans), lentils, and dried green peas (which are legumes, not vegetables). Soy/edamame are also good choices.

Make legumes a staple of your diet, second only to vegetables and fruits.

3. Nuts and Seeds

Nuts and seeds make for a great snack throughout the day,

but be careful not to eat too many as they are high in calories and fat (though it's healthy fat). Since reducing caloric intake is important, especially if weight loss is needed, consume nuts and seeds in moderation.

You can choose your favorite nuts and/or seeds, anything goes: peanuts (which are technically legumes), cashews, walnuts, almonds, macadamia nuts, pistachios, sunflower seeds, pumpkin seeds - anything you enjoy can be eaten in small quantities each day.

Just make sure that whatever you eat is not fried or roasted with added oils, or flavored with additional sugars or artificial seasonings. Stick to the plain, natural varieties.

4. Dairy Products

You can still include dairy in your diet, but not every day - and only certain types. While a bit of milk or low-fat yogurt each day is fine, it's important not to overdo it.

Here's what you should **never** consume (or only in tiny amounts once a month if you really miss the taste):

- Butter of any type

- Any cheese with more than 20% fat

- Full-fat yogurt (including Greek yogurt)

- High-fat milk varieties (full-fat milk, half-and-half, heavy cream, condensed milk, etc.)

- Any type of dairy with added sugars

So, what types of dairy can you have? There are still plenty of options:

- **Low-fat yogurt** (as long as it doesn't have added sugar - always read the ingredients!)

- **Low-fat milk** (again, make sure there's no added sugar)

- Various low-fat specialty yogurts like Skyr, Kefir, Ayran, etc.

- **Low-fat cheese** such as Cottage Cheese, Ricotta, or other varieties - both matured or not - as long as they have less than 20% fat.

Many people choose to avoid all dairy products, which is

completely fine. However, dairy is an important source of calcium, and I personally enjoy the taste. So, since there are still options, you can include them in your diet - and getting used to the low-fat varieties isn't difficult at all.

An important reminder: always read the labels and ensure there is no added sugar or other sweeteners. Unfortunately, in many countries, low-fat yogurt and other low-fat dairy products often have added sugar to compensate for the lack of fat, and added sugar is even worse than the fat itself!

I might sound like a broken record, but moderation is extremely important: when eating cheese, for example - even the low-fat varieties - aim for at most 50 grams per meal (and never have it daily).

5. Low-Fat Meat

You can consume low-fat meat a few times per week. I had periods when I ate some type of meat daily, so it's not the end of the world if you do too - but don't make it a habit.

You should only consume low-fat meats like chicken or

turkey breast, as well as lean fish such as cod, pollock, flounder, haddock, and so on.

Despite popular belief, you can still have some types of red meat - as long as you go for the leanest cuts. Here are some examples of red meats you can still consume:

- **Pork tenderloin:** This is the leanest part of pork and is similar in fat content to a skinless chicken breast (but with a bit more iron, so bonus points for pork).

- **Eye of round roast (aka round steak):** It's the leanest beef cut, with around 7% fat and plenty of iron.

- **Salmon:** Only go for the wild varieties. Although high in fat, it contains omega-3 fatty acids, which are essential for our health.

IMPORTANT: The red meats recommended above are acceptable, but they are also high in cholesterol, so they shouldn't be consumed often or in large quantities. If you eat meat three times per week, for example, limit red meat to just once.

Portion sizes should also be kept under control. A portion

of any type of meat should be between 85 grams to 125 grams (3 - 5 ounces), roughly the size of an adult's palm but cut thinly.

The only exception is with fish and seafood - if you choose the leanest varieties available, you can eat them more often in addition to other types of meat.

Always prepare meats by grilling, boiling, or roasting in the oven, with no added fats or sugars (including marinades made with sugars, honey, or anything similar). Add plenty of herbs for extra flavor and always pair them with a hearty side of vegetables and leafy greens salads.

6. Grains and Pseudocereals

You might remember this category from the "foods to avoid" section. While some grains should indeed be eliminated (such as white wheat, white rice, and highly processed grains), you can still consume other types in moderation.

Here are some options you can eat:

- **Whole wheat flour**
- **Whole grain flours:** Barley, Millet, Rye

- **Pseudocereals:** Quinoa, Amaranth, Chia, Buckwheat

- **Whole grain rice:** Brown, Black, Red, Wild, etc.

Bread: Ideally, you should cut bread out of your diet completely. If you're like me and find that difficult, try to limit yourself to a maximum of 2 slices of healthy, whole-wheat or whole-grain bread (without added sugar or other chemicals) per meal, or a keto bread replacement, including rye bread made with sourdough. However, keep your daily intake to a maximum of 3 slices. If you can manage some days without eating any bread, that's even better.

Make sure to read the ingredient list if you don't bake your own bread at home. Healthy bread only needs a few ingredients (flour, water, salt, and yeast). Avoid bread with added sugars, additives, flavorings, preservatives, and similar ingredients. If mixes of flour are used, ensure they are all whole wheat or whole grain.

Finding healthy bread in stores can be challenging, so it's often better to make your own at home. I purchased a bread maker for this purpose and am quite happy with it, so you might consider investing in one if you don't have time to bake manually. It doesn't taste as good, but at least you have an option.

Rice & Pasta: These are considered important parts of the Mediterranean diet but are, unfortunately, on our "don't eat" list in most cases. However, like the other grains and pseudocereals listed above, there are some healthier options available.

Typically, both rice and pasta are highly processed foods that provide a large amount of quickly absorbed carbs, which isn't ideal. This is especially true for white rice varieties and regular pasta.

However, you can still enjoy moderate amounts of healthier options. As mentioned earlier, brown, wild, or black rice can be consumed since it's not refined, meaning the carbs are absorbed more slowly. Plus, you get extra fiber and nutrients.

The same applies to pasta. There are varieties made from whole wheat flour and alternatives like lentils, chickpeas, or green pea pasta that might be suitable. Pasta replacements like konjac is also a viable alternative. Just make sure to read the ingredient list and look for lower amounts of carbs and higher amounts of fiber.

Remember that all these types of foods - whether we're talking about healthy, homemade bread, rye bread, wild rice, or whole wheat pasta - still contain plenty of carbs. So, keep portions small and eat them only occasionally.

Also, note that eating a portion of pasta or rice replaces one of your daily slices of bread.

7. Sugar & Sweetened Foods/Drinks

While it's true that sugars, like all carbohydrates, provide our bodies with energy, we should eliminate added sugar from our diet. You'll still get enough carbs from all the healthy foods you'll be eating, mainly from cereals, fruits, and vegetables.

Even though we've already discussed this, I must emphasize it again, as sugar is a major culprit in developing a fatty liver.

Stop eating sugar of any type! Stop adding sugar to your foods!

If you absolutely must add sweetness (though ideally, you shouldn't), reduce the amount to a quarter of what you'd normally use. Consider replacing white sugar with more natural alternatives like honey, maple syrup, or agave syrup. Even better, try to use safe sugar alternatives such as Stevia, sugar alcohols (erythritol, maltitol), or mashed fruits (like banana or apple puree) if you're baking. But the goal is to say no to sugar.

You'll need to eliminate all sorts of sweets found in stores, restaurants, and pastry shops: candies, cakes, chocolates, pastries, frozen desserts (ice cream, gelato, sorbet), milkshakes, and so on. These should no longer be consumed once you've been diagnosed with a fatty liver, even if you make them at home (if you add sugars).

All sweets are extremely harmful to our health. The high carb content in sweets is damaging, especially to the liver. Additionally, these sweets are often calorie bombs made of sugar and fat, with little nutritional value, which further underscores why you should avoid them.

While it's ideal to eliminate them entirely, I know how challenging it is. I had cheat days to combat dieting fatigue and it wasn't the end of the world. Aim for at most two cheat days per month early on, then once per week after reversing your fatty liver disease. However, it's crucial to keep foods with added sugars to a minimum, even during cheat days.

I also try to make my own desserts at home, using sugar alternatives or at least reducing the sugar in recipes by at least half (you'll find that they're still sweet and tasty!).

Sooner rather than later, you'll find yourself opting for less sweet and healthier options, and you'll start to find the sweets you once enjoyed overly sweet and unappealing. And yes, there are acceptable desserts you can find in specialty shops - just make sure to read the ingredient list!

Alternatives to Sugar

Raw Honey: It is sweet, natural, and tastes good. However, while it's healthier than white sugar, it still packs a lot of carbs (which essentially become sugar in your body), so consume it in moderation.

For instance, 100 grams of sugar contain 100 grams of carbs, while 100 grams of honey contain 82 grams of carbs. That's still a lot! However, the sugar in honey is absorbed more slowly than white sugar (which is good), and honey also has other nutrients that provide antioxidant, anti-inflammatory, and antimicrobial properties.

IMPORTANT: Honey becomes toxic if heated, so don't use it for cooking, baking, or frying (it's still safe to add to your tea or coffee or other warm beverages).

Maple Syrup: In my opinion, Maple Syrup is a better choice than honey for two reasons: it contains fewer sugars/carbs, and it is considered heat stable by most experts, therefore you can use it when cooking/baking.

Carbs: 100 grams of maple syrup have 67 grams of carbs, compared to 100 grams of sugar and 82 grams of honey. This makes it a better choice since we should always aim to keep carb intake as low as possible.

Stevia: Once considered a wonder sweetener because it's a zero-calorie sweetener (with no carbs), some recent studies have raised concerns about its safety. So definitely do your own research and decide if you should use it. I personally used it and still do, based on the fact that we have so few options anyway.

Some people also report a slightly metallic aftertaste with Stevia (though not everyone experiences this). Pure Stevia is 200 times sweeter than sugar, so adjust the quantity used accordingly. Make sure that you get pure Stevia, too: most of the products labelled as Stevia only have tiny amounts of this sweetener and plenty of other alternatives, not always healthy.

Erythritol: Another sweetener I used regularly, although it has come under scrutiny after a recent study suggested it might be linked to a higher risk of heart attack or stroke. I've since reduced my consumption but haven't completely eliminated it from my diet. I still consider it a valid option, though it's best to limit its use.

Note: Erythritol is a sugar alcohol, but despite the name, it has nothing to do with actual alcohol, meaning you can't get drunk from it, nor will you experience alcohol's side effects. It is nearly as sweet as regular sugar, with almost no calories and no effect on blood sugar.

By making these adjustments and being mindful of your choices, you can manage your sugar intake more effectively, which is crucial for reversing fatty liver disease.

8. What Is the Best Oil for Fatty Liver?

Before we start, it's important to reiterate: you should avoid eating any deep-fried foods, no matter what type of oil is used. Additionally, when preparing your meals, keep the amount of added oil to a minimum.

The one type of oil that is widely considered ideal for fatty liver is extra virgin olive oil (EVOO). Avocado oil is another good option, but it isn't necessarily better than EVOO.

Given that avocado oil is significantly more expensive, there's little reason to choose it over extra virgin olive oil, which is the only type of oil I've used since my diagnosis. If you can opt for cold-pressed, organic EVOO, it's even better, as it's considered the healthiest choice.

Olive oil is a staple of the Mediterranean Diet, known for its high content of unsaturated (healthy) fats, including polyunsaturated fats, and a wealth of antioxidants, which are excellent for liver health. Moreover, the healthy fats and antioxidants in EVOO appear to reduce the risk of cardiovascular disease, offering an additional benefit.

According to the US National Center for Biotechnology Information, extra virgin olive oil, particularly the first-pressed oil with maximum free acidity, contains an abundance of squalene and phenolic antioxidants, including simple phenols (hydroxytyrosol, tyrosol), aldehydic secoiridoids, flavonoids, and lignans (acetoxypinoresnol, pinoresinol). Notably, it has significantly higher concentrations of these antioxidants and squalene than other refined virgin and seed oils.

When purchasing olive oil, ensure you buy from a

reputable brand and store, as counterfeit extra virgin olive oil is, unfortunately, becoming more common.

Whenever possible, cook your own meals. This gives you complete control over the ingredients, including fat and sugar content.

I exclusively use extra virgin olive oil - but in very small amounts - mainly for salads. For most other dishes, I cook without using any oil or add just a tablespoon near the end of the cooking process. After a few days of eating this way, you'll likely find that your food still tastes delicious without the extra oil - I promise!

To help you on this journey, I've included a variety of recipes in a later chapter that will keep your diet as varied as possible. You can use these as a starting point to create your own combinations and cook your meals with confidence.

3.5.2 List of Foods You Can Eat Daily / Weekly

To make things even easier for you, here is a list with plenty of food types that are allowed if you follow this diet. I'm trying to create a complete list, but chances are that some foods are still left out. Do some research if you can't find a food listed below, looking mainly at the fat and carb content, as these are what matter the most: the lower the values, the better the food.

Also, you don't HAVE to eat all of these foods, nor have them as often as I recommend. But get familiarized with the list below, as these are all main ingredients that you can use and mix for your meals from now on.

Foods you can eat daily

FRUITS	VEGETABLES	OTHER
Apple	Artichoke	All herbs/spices (natural)
Apricot	Asparagus	Oats/Oatmeal

Avocado	Bell Peppers	Low fat milk (eg in coffee/tea)
Banana	Broccoli	Nuts & Nut butter
Berries	Brussels sprouts	Seeds
Cherries	Cabbage	Extra Virgin Olive Oil
Grapefruit	Cauliflower	Legumes
Kiwi	Celery	Chiar
Lemon	Cucumber	Quinoa
Orange	Greens	Amaranth
Papaya	Okra	Buckwheat
Pear	Onion	Coconut
Pineapple	Root vegetables (radish, beets, carrots, etc.)	Apple Cider Vinegar
Plum	Tomato	-
Pomello	Zucchini	-
Watermelon	All Peppers	-
Basically, all fruits in moderation.	All Sprouts	-

Foods you can eat weekly/bi-weekly

Grapes	Squashes	Shellfish (oysters, crabs, lobster, shrimp, etc)
Figs	Eggs	Olives
Eggplant	Low-fat dairy products (including low-fat cheese)	Tofu
Potatoes	Chicken/Turkey Breast	Sweet Corn
Sweet Potatoes	Pork Tenderloin	Salmon, Tuna, Mackerel (wild)
Whole Wheat Flour Products	Eye of round roast	Low-fat Fish (wild)
Whole Grain Flour Products	Honey, Maple Syrup (in tiny quantities)	Whole Rice (Brown, Black, Red, Wild)
Green Peas	Agave Syrup (small quantities)	Olives

3.5.3 How Many Times Per Day Should You Eat?

I recommend eating five times per day, in smaller portions. This is more of a guideline than a must-follow rule though: adapt it to your daily schedule, adapting the amount of calories at the end of the day to the number of meals you had.

For example, I usually eat six times each day, although sometimes I only stick to the three main meals only. But usually, smaller meals makes it easier to not feel hungry at all times. Here's what my daily eating routine looks like:

- **Breakfast**: As soon as I wake up, usually between 7 AM and 7:30 AM

- **Morning snack**: Around 10:30 AM

- **Lunch**: At 1 PM

- **Afternoon snack**: Around 4:30 PM

- **Dinner**: At 6 PM

- **Late snack**: At around 8 PM (not always—it's better without it!)

The late snack can be adjusted to fit your own situation. I

usually go to bed early, around 10 PM, which leaves me with about four hours of not eating before sleeping. If my dinner was light, I usually get hungry right before bed time.

Since extreme hunger can derail your progress, it's best to avoid letting it happen. That's why, if I find dinner was too light, I allow myself a small snack by 8 PM at the latest. This still gives my digestive system at least two hours to handle the food before I go to sleep.

However, I've been experimenting with eliminating the late snack by eating a slightly more substantial dinner. This seems to work well, as I finish my last meal of the day at 6 PM, which gives me at least 13 hours of fasting before breakfast. For those without other health issues, fasting is believed to provide additional benefits. So an extra win if you can do it!

3.5.4 How Much Should You Eat?

Without becoming obsessed about it, it's important to establish a daily calorie target and plan your meals around it. This is most important when you're starting the diet, as most of us are used to eating larger portions than we should - and that' without even considering the quality of the food we're eating.

Your portions should be small but still sufficient to offer proper nutrition. If you're used to eating large portions, don't immediately switch to tiny amounts, as this drastic change might be difficult to adapt to and could lead to frustration or, worse, giving up because it will seem unsustainable.

Instead, gradually reduce your portion sizes over the course of a month, cutting a bit more food every few days until you reach the target amount. Remember, you likely need to lose weight and maintain it afterward, so it's a lasting lifestyle change we're talking about - hence the extra care on how we do it.

In other words, don't rush the process! Start by gradually cutting back on portions so your body can adjust. For example, I now eat about half of what I used to before my diagnosis (and it's crazy to realize how much food I ate - food my body didn't need!). Even though it was difficult at first, even with the gradual reduction of portion sizes, I got used with it eventually. Now, years after making this change, I never feel hungry at the end of the meal. On the contrary - I feel better than ever and so will you!

The key is not to starve yourself to lose weight. Weight loss boils down to one principle: calorie deficit. It's as simple as that! A calorie deficit can be achieved in two ways only: eating less and/or increasing your physical activity.

So, if you need, let's say, 2,500 calories to maintain your current weight, reduce your daily intake to 2,000–2,200 calories. This will help you lose around half a kilogram (1.1 pounds) per week, which is considered a safe and sustainable rate of weight loss early on.

Eventually, you will hit a point where the 2,200 calories will be required to maintain your new weight. If you still need to lose more, gradually reduce your daily calories further until you reach your ideal weight. Afterward, maintain your caloric intake at a level that sustains your new weight.

Taking it slow gives you time to get used to smaller portions, making it easier to stick with in the long term. If you're currently eating 4,000 calories a day and suddenly drop to 2,000, it will be a huge shock to your system and much harder to sustain on the long term. So take it slower!

Also, consider incorporating high-volume, low-calorie foods, especially at the beginning. These foods allow you to eat larger portions while still consuming fewer calories and maintaining a healthy diet. Examples include zucchini, cucumber, leafy greens, and watermelon, among many others.

You can use these strategies during your transition period, but the ultimate goal is to train your body to adapt to smaller portion sizes over time.

You Will Lose Weight Naturally, in a Healthy Way

When I started following the diet recommended above, I weighed 210 lbs (I'm 5'11"). I naturally lost weight without any extra exercise and without feeling starved.

I dropped to 190 lbs in three months, which is why I didn't initially add exercise to my routine: you don't want to lose weight too quickly, as it could put extra strain on your liver.

However, it's important to note that this fatty liver diet is not specifically a weight loss diet. In my case, the weight loss happened because I had been eating large portions of unhealthy foods. Switching to smaller portions and completely healthy foods helped me lose weight and maintain that weight over the years. I was amazed at how much our eating habits impact our weight!

Eventually, you'll reach a point where weight loss will slow down or plateau. This is when you should start incorporating exercise into your routine if you still need to lose weight.

From personal experience, I can say this usually happens after about three months of following the recommended Mediterranean diet.

Exercise is extremely important, so try to add something

extra to your routine, even if it's just walking 10,000 steps a day. More intense exercises like jogging or going to the gym are even better - they take less time than walking, providing the same benefits in terms of calories burned. Some fitness experts also consider that more intense exercising is better for your general health that slower paced types.

So the higher the intensity, the better. Aim to exercise at least three times per week, ideally every day. If you're out of shape, start slow and gradually increase the intensity every few days or sessions. We'll discuss exercising for fatty liver in more detail in a later chapter, but I wanted to briefly touch on it now.

The main goal of this diet isn't just to lose weight, but to completely change your lifestyle. This isn't a diet you follow for a month or two or until you reverse your fatty liver, and then to go back to your old habits. This is your new approach to food. This is how you live from now on!

3.5.5 What to Drink?

When managing a fatty liver, your drinking options are relatively limited, with plain water being the best choice. However, drinking only water can get boring quickly, so you'll need some alternatives to keep things interesting. Fortunately, there are plenty of options to keep your beverage selection varied.

First, let's recap the things you SHOULD NOT drink anymore:

- **Alcohol of any type.**

- **Any drink with added sugar or sugar alternatives** that significantly increase the carbohydrate content.

- **Fruit juices** (even those labeled as 100% fruit), including homemade juices, because juicing removes most of the nutrients while concentrating the sugars, making them almost as unhealthy as sodas.

After eliminating the above, you still have plenty of options. Here are some beverages you can enjoy daily, in addition to plain water:

- **Sparkling water**

- **Lemon water** (Add one teaspoon of freshly squeezed lemon or lime per glass. You can enhance it with cucumber slices, mint leaves, or other herbs, but no sugar.)

- **Coffee** (Ideally, drink it black, but you can add some low-fat milk.)

- **Tea & herbal tea** (Choose varieties without artificial flavors or sweeteners.)

- **Smoothies** (These aren't technically drinks, but you can enjoy them as a snack or meal.)

Flavored water falls into a gray area. You can have it occasionally as a treat, but always make sure to pick varieties without added sugars and ideally without artificial flavors.

3.5.6 Is This an Easy Diet to Follow?

I'll be honest: it's not easy. For me, it was a drastic change, and cutting all those unhealthy foods from my diet was challenging. There were cravings, and there were times when I broke down and ate too much, feeling miserable afterward.

So, you'll probably find it at least a bit difficult too - there's no need to sugarcoat it. Be prepared!

Fortunately, the diet itself becomes enjoyable after a while, allowing you to eat a wide variety of dishes. The most challenging parts (at least for me) were reducing portion sizes, cutting down on fats, and especially eliminating sugars. If you don't already have a sweet tooth, you'll find it much easier.

I used to always have around a chocolate bar or some candy before being diagnosed, and it was tough to stop that habit. Looking back, this was probably one of the main reasons why I developed a fatty liver in the first place... so good riddance!

But you'll soon get used to having an apple for dessert instead of sugary sweets, so it's not a never-ending struggle (though the first two or three weeks will be the toughest!).

Interestingly, if you taste any fried or fatty food a few months after switching to this diet, you'll likely find it unpleasant and overly greasy. I was surprised to realize that just a few months earlier, I used to consider that kind of food delicious.

I believe you'll start seeing major improvements after the first month of following this diet, and by around the six-month mark, you'll feel like a new person - slimmer, healthier, and full of energy. The pain under your right rib should be gone, along with any other regular symptoms. It's time enough, for some people, to even fully reverse their fatty liver.

It's important to remember, though, that it probably took years, if not decades, of unhealthy eating and lack of exercising to get where you are now. You can't expect things to change in a week or even a month. Healing takes time in this case - but fortunately, not the same among of years or decades if you do it right.

Some people who followed these guidelines reversed their

fatty liver as quickly as a couple of months. Some needed six months. I needed 18 months, for example, while others might need a bit more. It's important to stick to the diet, no matter how long it takes, and get it reversed!

And after you reverse your fatty liver, continue to stick to this Mediterranean diet. Don't return to old habits, as your fatty liver will definitely come back if you do. Stick to eating healthy, follow this balanced diet, and enjoy being healthy!

3.6 How to Beat Dieting Fatigue & Stick to Your Weight Loss Plan

If I had to pick one thing that prevents most people with fatty liver from reversing it, I'd say it's sticking to the diet. This is absolutely normal - it's a major lifestyle change, and it's not easy!

All of the emails I receive from people with NAFLD/MASLD who are struggling to reverse it have a common theme: they get sidetracked. They start off well, but after a while, they allow themselves a reward. Or Christmas comes. Or Thanksgiving. Or another important celebration where food is plentiful and delicious, and it's difficult to say no.

Does this sound familiar? It sure does to me! But don't worry - the truth is that most people go through this phase. I went through it too, but I still reversed my fatty liver. The most important thing is to get back on track as soon as you realize you're straying from what you should be doing.

As soon as I got the "all clear" from my doctor, I decided to offer myself a "small" treat. After all, I was healed and I deserved a reward, right? We celebrated with cake that day. During the weekend, we had pizza.

One month later, I had gained 11 pounds (5 kilograms). My liver had just been healed, and there I was, losing control and being stupid again, risking all the progress ove the past year and a half for food I honestly no longer enjoyed as much as I did before starting my diet. That's when I realized I had to stop immediately. It was as difficult as the first three weeks of dieting were - but equally important.

The lifestyle changes we're making, especially the new diet, have to be permanent. We have to accept and embrace these changes forever. It might sound bad, but it's not, because nothing is more important than staying healthy.

So, how do you beat dieting fatigue? How do you handle getting sidetracked?

My best friend since being diagnosed with fatty liver, and

what I recommend you as well, is a deceptively simple item that helps you stay motivated: a scale.

Get a scale, measure your weight daily, and keep a diary of your weight!

This is more powerful than you can imagine! It's essential to measure your weight daily - not weekly, not every few days, not every now and then, but EVERY. SINGLE. DAY.

Check your weight daily, even after splurging on a Saturday evening when you couldn't say no to that pizza! Monitoring your weight daily will not only keep you motivated, but it will also teach you a lot about what to eat, what to avoid, and how various (unhealthy) foods affect your body and especially your weight.

If you've just been diagnosed with a fatty liver, get a scale as soon as possible - it will motivate you even more to stay focused! I started using this method about a week after my diagnosis, following my doctor's recommendation, and it was incredibly helpful.

Early on, if you're overweight, you'll lose weight quickly when switching to my recommended diet. Watching those numbers drop daily will make you feel amazing! You'll see your progress recorded on that piece of paper - or any app you use for that purpose - day by day, week by week. Each new number will be lower than the last. You'll see the results of your hard work, feel better, and have every reason to keep going.

You'll also see the effects of stepping off track. You'll learn that splurging on pizza, soda, and a "small" dessert can mean gaining 2 extra pounds overnight - pounds that will take at least a couple of days to lose. You'll see what a chocolate bar can do to your body and what eating a lettuce salad for dinner instead of steak will mean. You'll learn what to eat, and you'll do your best to stay on track!

This method has helped me tremendously on multiple occasions. I started at 210 pounds (95kg) and lost weight quickly during the first few of months. I was proud of myself and loved seeing the numbers I recorded. Eventually, I reached my ideal weight of 165 pounds (75kg).

Then I went on vacation.

I didn't carry my scale, obvious, and also promised myself some treats as long as I ate healthier than I used to before my diagnosis. I was on vacation, after all! I had reversed my fatty liver, was in great shape, and everything seemed fine. What could go wrong?

Well... this happened: when I returned home after seven blissful days, I had gained 15 pounds (almost 7 kilograms)! I still looked good, and my overall weight wasn't bad at all. But the real problem was that I had no idea I had gained so much weight! If the scale hadn't told me, I would've been content with the outcome and maybe, on the next vacation, done the same and added 15 more pounds. Then I might've said yes to extra cake, more burgers, and pizzas, undoing my progress.

But the scale told me otherwise. The numbers I had written on my weight tracker before the vacation told me otherwise. So I started working on losing weight again - much slower than before - but I eventually got back to my ideal weight. The scale and those numbers keep you on track. They keep you motivated!

There's one more important thing to realize: getting sidetracked, gaining extra pounds, and losing focus for a while is natural. It happens to everyone. It's not the end of the world!

But it can be the end of the world if you make it a habit.

Did you eat a hearty meal at a party? It happens. But don't have dessert just because you've already moved away from your plan. Failure is something you choose, not something that randomly happens. Make the choice to eat that hearty meal and own it. But make it a singular event, not a new rule!

The same goes for sweets and anything else you shouldn't have. Did you grab a candy bar from the box, but there are nine more left? You don't have to eat them all just because you ate one! It's understandable if you ate one after months of dieting, but there's no excuse if you choose to keep doing it, although you know you shouldn't.

Most people I've talked to admitted that one thing led to another: they first allowed themselves to eat a big pizza at a party and felt bad for doing so. But then came the cake, so they decided to eat that too, reasoning that the harm was already done.

Then, the next day, feeling miserable because they cheated the other day, ate some ice cream... and so on.

But this is wrong! We're just making up excuses to justify doing what we're not supposed to. We know - or should know - very well that eating a whole pizza is bad. But it's not as bad as eating an entire pizza AND having some cake afterward. It's not as bad as eating another pizza the next day because there are leftovers from others...

One of the most important things when getting sidetracked is to accept your slip-up, acknowledge that you lost a battle, but then recover to win the war!

Here are some other tips and tricks for beating dieting fatigue. Use as many as needed to stick to your schedule and reach your goal: reversing fatty liver and staying healthy afterward!

1. Have a Cheat Day

I allow myself to cheat once a month and on special occasions (holidays, birthdays), which usually means I cheat, on average, about once every three weeks or so.

When I cheat, I eat things I wouldn't normally eat, but without going overboard. I'm not jumping into fries and burgers, with a large milkshake on the side, but I might have a few slices of pepperoni pizza or something that's greasy or sweet (but one thing, not all of them!).

Cheat, but in moderation! Eat a burger, but nothing else. Eat a cake, but nothing else. It's even better if you can cook your cheat foods at home and use less fat and sugar - they're still tasty and good, but healthier than restaurant-bought options.

Once you're on the right track with your diet and especially after reversing your fatty liver disease, I believe these cheat days are vital for the long-term success of your dieting. Just make sure you don't overdo it and turn cheating into a habit!

2. Know What Signs Your Body Is Sending

After all these years, I've learned to recognize the warning signs - those fatty liver symptoms - easily now.

When I feel bloated almost daily, notice my belly starting to look full and unattractive again, and begin to feel less comfortable in my skin, including that familiar upper right side pain, I know I'm slipping back into old habits.

These signs are my body's way of saying, "Stop, you fool!" It's a reminder that I'm harming myself again, and if I keep going, I'll end up where I was before - or maybe worse. But now, I recognize these signals. They're my cue to stop the bad habits and get back on track. So learn to listen to your body and act accordingly!

3. Think About Your Loved Ones

When I was first diagnosed and learned how this disease could progress into something really nasty, I started crying. I thought I was going to die, and all I could think about was my family, especially my then 1-year-old son. I promised myself that

I would never let myself get into that situation again.

He's 11 now, as I write this book, and I want to cherish every second I spend by his side - and hopefully do so for many years to come.

Every day, I remind myself of that moment when I felt like my world had ended and I prayed to God for one more chance to enjoy more time with my family.

I cried like a terrified child, and I don't ever want to go back there. I have to fight for what I promised myself - and what I ultimately achieved. It's not worth that extra sip of unhealthy soda or any other indulgence that could jeopardize my health. Do the same, do it constantly, and stay focused!

4. Check Your Weight Daily

As I've mentioned before, you need a scale to check your weight daily. Write it down (piece of paper, weight tracker, app - whatever works for you). This way, you can easily keep your weight under control and notice when you're starting to slip back into old, unhealthy habits.

5. Keep Yourself Motivated

It's true that there are countless temptations around us, that our own minds can work against us, and that loved ones may still enjoy fries, greasy foods, ice cream, cake, candy, and so on. But living is about more than just filling your belly!

Life is more than eating, and there are so many other ways to enjoy it! The best way to enjoy life is to know that you are healthy. Fight for your health and never give up! Overcome these obstacles, leave them behind, and fight for your well-being! You're fighting for happiness - and that should be enough to keep you going!

Watch motivational videos on YouTube, even if they aren't related to fatty liver. Just do a search for "motivational video" and select one or more from the results. You will eventually find one that ticks with you and gives you that extra push to keep going.

One video that I always listen to when I need some motivation is titled "Hard Times ► Motivational Video." Simply copy and paste this into the YouTube search bar, and you'll find it! If this particular one doesn't work for you, there are plenty of others online. Find one that does and watch it regularly for a massive boost of confidence and motivation!

6. Keep the Unhealthy Stuff Away

Remove all the distractions that can steer you off course: it's easier to avoid sugary drinks, high-fat biscuits, or candy bars if they're not around you.

In my case - and probably for most people - it's difficult to completely eliminate temptations, especially if you have an 11-year-old around.

But I have a pact with my wife: she hides all the "goodies," and only she knows where they are. Of course, I know where the bad things are - but it's a shelf I never check. My family is supportive enough to eat as little of those unhealthy items in my presence as possible, so it's easier to stay away from them.

The harder it is to access unhealthy stuff, the less likely you are to indulge.

There was a time when we kept our son's candy in a jar on

the table. After a couple of weeks, I realized that I was eating more of it than he was. (And probably he was also eating more than he would've otherwise, simply because you always bumped into it). After moving it to a less obvious spot, it became much easier to resist - I haven't eaten a single candy from that jar since!

So keep all the unhealthy stuff away. Ideally, don't have any at home, but if you due because of your loved ones, make sure you don't have easy access to that food.

3.7 Exercising to Reverse Fatty Liver Disease

While diet is the most crucial factor in reversing fatty liver, exercise is also essential for a complete turnaround. Incorporating regular physical activity into your life is part of the new, healthier you.

You don't need to hit the gym every day or aim for breaking world records, though that certainly wouldn't hurt. However, you do need to include some form of exercise and physical activity in your routine, and the sooner you start, the better.

It's also important to monitor how quickly you're losing weight. Ideally, you shouldn't lose more than about 2 pounds (1 kilogram) per week - although losing a bit more is not the end of the world.

Initially, this may happen from dietary changes alone, as it was my case. Eventually, though, you may hit a plateau or experience a slowdown in weight loss. That's when incorporating various forms of exercise becomes mandatory.

If you're not physically fit or haven't exercised in a while, start slowly. There's no need to push yourself to exhaustion just to quit a few moments later because it feels too difficult. It's only difficult if you make it so.

You just need to start somewhere, even if you're significantly overweight and out of shape. For example, begin by walking for 10 minutes per day at a moderate pace, three days in a row. Then increase your walking time to 15 minutes for the next three days. After that, try walking 20 minutes each day for a week. Gradually increase your speed and, if possible, the duration of your walks.

Your goal should be to walk briskly for at least one hour per day, but there's no need to rush. Think of it as a marathon - something you'll continue for the rest of your life. So it's okay if it takes you a month to reach that goal!

In many cases, just walking for an hour a day is enough if you're otherwise moderately active and not spending the rest of the day sitting on a couch. But you can and should aim for more!

Especially if you're younger or more physically fit, your goal should include more intense aerobic exercise and/or strength training to lose weight and keep your body healthy.

I decided to join a gym - and that's what I recommend to those who can't stick to a self-imposed schedule. I tried creating a workout schedule at home, but I often found myself getting distracted, finding all sorts of excuses and skipping my sessions. That's a mistake because nothing is more important than getting healthy and staying healthy! But it happened.

Signing up for the gym helped me stay organized. Paying for a membership gave me an extra reason to go as often as possible - I didn't want to waste the money. Plus, it established a routine. I treated it like a job: between 4-6 PM, I was at the gym. Of course, you should find the best time that works for you, even if it's just 60 minutes or even less.

But creating this routine became a natural part of my schedule, something I knew I had to do. Although my goal was to go to the gym daily, I ended up going three times a week. The rest of the time, I exercised at home whenever I could, and I made sure to walk at least 8,000 steps each day (usually ending up with 12,000 to 15,000).

Yes, it would be ideal to go to the gym daily - if you can do it, that's perfect. But don't worry if you can't - even three times a week is good and most likely a lot better than you were doing before.

I also recommend choosing a personal trainer if possible. Make sure to get an experienced one and inform them that your goal is to lose weight gradually to heal your liver (as they often push for fast, extreme weight loss). A personal trainer can adjust your exercise intensity based on your fitness level and weight loss goals. They will also keep you motivated and help you stick to your gym schedule. Just be sure to start slow and gradually increase the intensity.

Ultimately, it depends on how much motivation you need from others and how much you can do on your own. I am self-employed, so it's easier for me to create a schedule and stick to it because I've been doing that for years. But even if you need some extra help, it's easily attainable - don't be afraid or ashamed to ask for it.

If a personal trainer and the gym aren't your thing, you can always try something else. You could find some physically active friends and set up training sessions with them, or you could join groups to find jogging partners, go to dancing classes or anything similar. The only thing keeping you from exercising is yourself. So don't sabotage your quest for health - just start!

Once you do, it's essential to stick to your program! It doesn't matter if it's raining, hot, or freezing (as long as it's not actually unsafe outside), if you don't feel like doing it, or if a friend wants to meet during your exercise time. You stick to your program because that's what's making you healthy!

You don't stop going to your job because the weather isn't great, because there's something nice on TV, or because your favorite shop has a sale. Or because you don't feel like it. These reasons shouldn't stop you from exercising either, especially since it benefits you on so many levels!

Note: If you have other health issues (like hypertension), exercising in extreme weather might not be advisable. Make sure to discuss your options with your doctor based on your overall health and decide what's the best approach for you.

3.8 Friends & Family: They Can Make or Break It for You

I keep emphasizing that diet is the most important factor in reversing your fatty liver. It goes hand in hand with exercise, which is the second most important component.

But other factors - some that seem to have no apparent effect and others that may seem too small to matter - can also play a significant role in either helping or hindering your efforts to reverse fatty liver disease.

One aspect that we might not give enough credit to (or pay enough attention to), but which is extremely important, is managing your interactions with family and friends, and ensuring they understand the seriousness of your condition and your need for support.

In the end, it's friends and family who can either greatly aid or severely hinder your progress in reversing fatty liver. Small things matter: when you're on the edge of the cliff, it only takes a small push to send you over...

In this case, the "edge" might be a burger, a huge slice of cake, a glass of wine, or something similar, and the "push" could be a friend or family member insisting you indulge.

Since family can be a bit more challenging to navigate, let's start by looking at your social circle. In theory, it's straightforward: stop spending time with "friends" who don't understand or respect your new lifestyle. Yes, it's incredibly difficult in most cases, and it can hurt at first, but ask yourself this: do you want to keep your drinking buddy, or do you want to live longer and stay close to the people who truly love you and want the best for you?

Before being diagnosed with a fatty liver disease, I was socially active and often went out with different groups of friends. I had a pretty solid social circle, and having fun usually meant going out to a pub and drinking too much, or meeting up at a friend's house (or mine) and drinking similar amounts, but on a budget. Yes, we had a great time, but what I didn't realize at the time was that my body was suffering.

NOTE: Even though my diagnosis - and yours - was "non-alcoholic fatty liver disease," as we've already discussed, alcohol doesn't help at all. On the contrary - it causes plenty of harm!

Then my doctor confirmed I had fatty liver disease, and I had to make a choice: either continue what I was doing and risk severe health consequences, or stop. So I stopped.

It was a temporary pause. For a solid month (maybe even longer), I stopped going out entirely to avoid temptation. But eventually, I wanted to see my friends again and enjoy a night out (minus the alcohol and unhealthy food). So I went out.

All of my close friends already knew about my health issues, the new diet I had to follow, and especially the fact that I couldn't drink alcohol anymore. Most of them understood. Many said nothing when I ordered sparkling water. Some even chose not to drink alcohol when we met up (kudos to these friends!). And we still had a great time together - something I didn't think was possible without having a few drinks to loosen up! That's

135

probably just the kind of nonsense we've been led to believe by companies to keep us hooked on their products.

But I digress. The truth is, not all my friends were as understanding or supportive. Some simply couldn't understand or accept my need to stop drinking alcohol or eat a healthier diet. They would say things like, "What, you mean you'll never drink again? Like, EVER? That's impossible!"

When we went out, they constantly tried to convince me to have a drink. It was as if they had something to gain from it. They tried everything - from buying drinks for me without asking, to various forms of manipulation, even guilt-tripping.

When they visited, they would always bring alcohol and were upset or offended when I refused to drink. It didn't matter that it was for my own well-being, that alcohol would harm my liver and potentially undo months of hard work aimed at improving my health and life.

Unfortunately, we live in a society where many people no longer prioritize the well-being of others. With instant gratification so readily available, some start to believe that anything others do, which doesn't align with their own values, needs, or wants, is somehow offensive.

Those are the "friends" I stopped seeing. It was difficult because, despite their behavior, I had great relationships with most of them, and I had known some since childhood. But I realized I didn't need that kind of influence in my life.

The toxic people. The ones who wouldn't stop until they got their way. And I wasn't about to give them the chance to succeed - especially not when my health was on the line.

Because, even though I consider myself strong-willed, there's always the possibility that, under the right circumstances, I might say yes. A special occasion, a bad mood, or even an exceptionally good one could lead me to say, "OK, just one sip," or "OK, I'll have dessert today." It's hard enough to resist these temptations on my own without added pressure - so why make things even harder for myself?

A friend is not truly a friend if they try to hurt you. When

137

they can't understand that your well-being is more important than their misguided ideas of "having fun" or "feeling good," or the personal goals they've set for themselves (some even made it their mission to see me drink again), they need to be removed from your life.

I wasn't an alcoholic, and none of my friends were either, even though my story might sound like that was the case. So don't think this can't happen to you or that you'll be able to handle it. It most likely will happen, and you'll have to remove these negative influences from your life. If they can't accept the new you, they don't deserve to be part of your life.

And this is not just about alcohol. If they bring pizza or unhealthy snacks over, if they visit and always bring soda/soft drinks, desserts or anything that you shouldn't have, it's just as bad.

Most people don't understand how hard it is to stick to a diet and deal with all the restrictions that come with it. Many will say it's impossible, that you'll eventually give up. These are also the people you don't need in your life. You need support, not added pressure. Make sure you remind them of this, and if they don't accept it, cut them off your list of friends or see them as little as possible.

It's your life. It's your health. Nothing is more important than that - especially not so-called friends who knowingly try to sabotage your efforts to become healthy and remain that way.

Friends are relatively easy to distance yourself from. But things become more complicated when it's a family member who struggles to accept your new lifestyle. We don't choose our family, and sometimes it can be hard for them to understand or adjust.

Personally, I had an especially hard time getting my mother to understand one key thing: that I no longer eat sugar. We met often, as we live in the same city, and we have a great relationship overall, but she always insisted on making something sweet for me to "try" when I visited. She would say, "There's no sugar in these cookies, try them!"

And I did, enjoying them - only for her to eventually admit she had added "just a little" sugar because otherwise, they wouldn't taste as good. Naturally, this upset me, and I eventually stopped eating anything she made.

Was she offended? Yes, at first. But I didn't let things escalate because I decided to take a different approach - one I strongly recommend to you as well.

Later that year, I organized a family meeting with all my close relatives.

I gathered everyone at my house and printed a large photo comparing a healthy liver to a fatty liver (it's easy to find online). I showed them the disturbing image and explained my situation, stressing the importance of sticking to my new diet in order to regain my health. I asked for their support and explained that this was much harder for me than it was for them. Thankfully, they understood. All it took was an honest conversation and a shocking image. But as long as it worked, I was happy with the result!

In fact, it went so well that my mother not only stopped lying about the ingredients in her cooking, but she also chose to follow a similar diet, cutting out added sugar and unhealthy fats. It was a significant change that she made not only to support me but also to improve her own health. Today, 10 years later, her blood work looks better than it has in decades, even though she doesn't follow as strict a diet as I do. And she's in her 70s!

Two years after that family meeting and several months after I had successfully reversed my fatty liver, I took my mother out to a restaurant to share some important news. It felt like a cause for celebration, so I considered ordering dessert. But when I called the waiter, my mother made a bit of a scene, not letting me order the said dessert. Initially, I felt embarrassed but in the end I didn't order anything.

Looking back, I realize it was the right decision. More importantly, it was my mother - a person who used to offer me things I shouldn't eat because she didn't fully understand my condition - who helped me say no and stick to my diet. It made me realize that sticking to a plan - whether it's a diet or a new way of living - is much easier when you have supportive people around you.

Yes, it was embarrassing at the time. A fit, adult man not ordering dessert because his mother intervened. But that moment helped me stay healthy, and nothing is more important than that.

In the end, make sure your family and friends understand what you're going through and accept your new lifestyle. Help them realize how important their support is - don't hesitate to ask for it directly, as this will motivate at least some to truly take care of you. Often, a clear, direct conversation can make them realize the seriousness of your condition and how much sticking to your plan matters to you.

So, don't be afraid to tell your friends and family about your health problem, and most importantly, don't hesitate to ask for their support. You'll find that when you need it the most, they'll be there for you.

3.9 Dealing with Stress

Stress can be a contributing factor to multiple health-related problems, including fatty liver disease. Various studies show a direct correlation between high stress levels and liver health issues.

I also believe that my own high stress levels were one of the direct or indirect causes of my fatty liver (along with other health problems), and managing stress played a key role in reversing my condition and getting my health back on track.

When you're stressed and feeling down, everything seems impossible, including the task of reversing your fatty liver - and especially dieting. While it's perfectly normal to feel overwhelmed after a diagnosis, you must not let this become the norm. Do not accept defeat, and do not let stress take over your life!

Stress comes at us from all directions: problems at work, issues at home, changes in weather, bad news - so many things pile up daily to increase our stress levels, bombarding us like we're in a constant battle. And controlling stress is another crucial element when it comes to healing your liver.

For example, I'm a stress eater - when I get extremely stressed after a tough day, I tend to eat for comfort, even though I know it's bad for my liver and overall health. It's something I've struggled with since forever, and although I've tried different ways to manage it, it hasn't been easy.

However, I am doing my best to keep things under control. Stress management techniques work differently for everyone, so I encourage you to do a bit of research to find what works for you. And of course, it's always a good idea to consult a professional.

Whether it's talking to yourself and giving yourself pep talks in the mirror (which oddly works for me), listening to music, practicing yoga, doing breathing exercises, meditating, reading a good book, going out for a run, or something else, try different methods until you find what helps you manage stress. Then make it a habit - use it regularly to keep your stress under control. It's much easier to fight fatty liver disease with the right mindset!

I can't stress enough (no pun intended!) how important it is to stay positive, to reduce stress as much as possible, to build your confidence, and to take time for yourself.

Do whatever it takes to smile every day, enjoy life, and appreciate the amazing opportunity you've been given: the chance to start over, become a better person, and get healthy. Encourage yourself and celebrate the progress you've made in your journey to reverse fatty liver. I guarantee that you will have all the reasons to be happy when you will start seeing the results of your new approach to eating and living!

Look at your fatty liver from a different perspective: not as a terrible health problem that stops you from enjoying your favorite foods or wine, but as an opportunity to try something new and grow into a healthier, better version of yourself.

Being healthy is one of the greatest gifts you can give to yourself and your loved ones, and that's exactly what you're doing! Always remember: your health and well-being are more valuable than a burger, a glass of wine, or a slice of cake.

It's all about the positive thinking here. It's all about looking at the bright side of life. Surrounding yourself with shiny, happy people. Start doing more of what you enjoy and less of what you don't. Take action! Find a new hobby if you don't have one and let it take over, enjoy it, live it, make it happen!

As difficult as it might seem to be, stop seeing the negative people, the energy leechers, the ones that make everything more difficult. Take breaks and spend some time alone if that is what you want - or more with your family if you so prefer. Free your mind of all bad things and feed it with positive thoughts. This helps tremendously and you will have a so much better life if you manage to do it!

4. Supplements & Other Natural Methods to Help You Reverse Fatty Liver Disease

I'm not someone who avoids taking medications prescribed by a doctor - I always have, and I always will, if advised by a professional, and I recommend everyone to do exactly as their doctor instructs them.

However, fatty liver disease is a condition that, in most cases - if not all - can and will be treated simply by changing your diet and exercising, and sticking to those changes.

While there are now some medications that either directly or indirectly help manage and even reverse fatty liver disease (more on this in a later chapter), it's crucial to remember that you still need to change your diet and incorporate more physical activity into your daily routine for long-time success. This is important because many people mistakenly believe they can just take a pill and solve their problem.

For this reason, I'm not particularly enthusiastic about

recommending any natural supplements, pills, herbal remedies, or homeopathic treatments as a way to battle fatty liver disease. Personally, I believe that most supplements, cleanses, and "remedies" won't be as effective as the two key strategies I've emphasized repeatedly: proper dieting and regular exercise.

That said, despite my reservations, I did try various supplements and natural remedies over the years, many of which were recommended by liver specialists or other healthcare professionals. Since studies indicate that, at the very least, these supplements do no harm - but hopefully they help speed up your recovery 0 I want to share my experiences with two of the most commonly suggested options: Milk Thistle and Apple Cider Vinegar.

I took both at different times and in various quantities (and other supplements too, but I believe these two are enough for most). While I can't say with 100% certainty that they helped me reverse my fatty liver disease, I know they didn't cause any harm since I eventually healed my liver. And since many people claim these supplements can be beneficial, I think they're worth discussing, so you can decide for yourself if you should take them or not.

4.1 Milk Thistle

Of all the dietary supplements claimed to help reverse fatty liver disease, Milk Thistle is probably the one mentioned most often

What is Milk Thistle? It's a plant scientifically known as *Silybum marianum* (nothing silly about it, though!), from the Asteraceae family. It has red to purple flowers and shiny pale green leaves with white veins, and it's been used for thousands of years to improve liver function and cleanse the liver.

I understand that some people are skeptical about plant-based medicines (and I've been one of them), but in this case, you might want to reconsider.

Not only has Milk Thistle been used for over 2,000 years as a natural remedy for liver diseases, but recent studies suggest that it may indeed have beneficial effects on the liver. When science backs up tradition, I'm ready to trust it!

Milk Thistle extract is commonly prescribed for treating mushroom poisoning, alcoholic cirrhosis, chronic hepatitis, drug-

and alcohol-induced liver damage, acute viral hepatitis, as well as fatty liver disease (NAFLD/MASLD). Many doctors consider it the most important supplement for maintaining a healthy liver.

Numerous studies (the U.S. National Library of Medicine and the National Institutes of Health report over 400) have shown that Milk Thistle has beneficial effects on the liver, with its active ingredient, silibinin (silybin), having hepatoprotective (antihepatotoxic) properties that protect liver cells against toxins.

In plain English, Milk Thistle appears to have a positive effect on the liver, helping to reduce ALT and AST levels, as well as fat and toxins accumulated in the liver.

The best part is that it rarely has any side effects. So, at worst, you may see no change from taking Milk Thistle supplements. But if the claims about its regenerative effects on damaged liver cells are true, then you stand to gain a lot.

Even though I can't say with 100% certainty that Milk Thistle will improve your liver health - since some studies suggest it may do no more than a placebo - I decided to take these supplements, especially since my hepatologist recommended them.

When deciding what type of Milk Thistle supplement to take for fatty liver disease, you should always consult your doctor. In my case, my doctor recommended a high dose (apparently, silybin is not easily absorbed by the human body) in the form of gel capsules (1,000 mg).

I took one pill in the morning every day for three months. After a one-month break, I resumed the treatment for another three months. This approach is generally considered safe, and I was already feeling a lot better after about 2.5 months of use.

I must repeat, though: I can't be certain whether it was the supplements, the diet and exercise, or a combination of all three that improved my condition. But I did feel better and my health improved, so at the very least, the supplements didn't hurt.

In conclusion, Milk Thistle is one of the few supplements I consider worth taking when trying to reverse fatty liver disease.

4.2 Apple Cider Vinegar

For years, apple cider vinegar (ACV) has been associated with reversing fatty liver, and many people who consume ACV or take it as a supplement swear by its beneficial effects. There is also scientific evidence showing that it helps reduce fat in the body, making it the second supplement I recommend.

However, "supplement" might not be the best word to use, because you can easily and naturally include ACV in your diet rather than taking it as a pill - something I recommend doing. This is what I did, and it seems it was a good approach.

How Does Apple Cider Vinegar Work?

There are many benefits to taking ACV for NAFLD or simply incorporating it into your daily diet. Here are some of the key benefits (according to Dr. Oz's website):

– Reduces blood sugar levels
– Lowers insulin levels, encouraging fat burning
– Improves metabolism function
– Reduces fat levels and helps burn fat

These are all great benefits for people with fatty liver, providing an additional tool to help reverse the condition as quickly as possible. The good news is that, apart from anecdotal evidence, numerous studies support these claims.

How to Take Apple Cider Vinegar for Fatty Liver

Before we talk about how to take ACV, it's important to note that you should aim for organic, raw, and unfiltered apple cider vinegar to ensure you're getting the full range of benefits. The price is a bit higher, but a bottle usually lasts about a month, so keep that in mind.

Here are a few ways you can take apple cider vinegar, so choose the one that works best for you:

1. The Traditional Method:

The most common way is to take it as a medicine every morning before eating. Mix one tablespoon (around 15ml) in a glass of warm water, stir well, and drink.

The taste isn't great, which is why some people add a bit of honey. I don't recommend this due to the fact that you're adding unnecessary carbs, but if you can't drink it otherwise, keep the honey to a minimum (no more than half a teaspoon).

Since vinegar is acidic, it may cause problems for those with acid reflux, gastritis, or similar conditions. As an alternative, you can take one of the many ACV pills out there.

2. During Meals:

A more natural way to consume ACV is by drinking the same amount (one tablespoon in a glass of water) during meals. This allows you to wash it down and continue eating.

You can also reduce the water content to half a glass. I personally believe this is a better option as it may help minimize some of the immediate side effects, and some fatty liver experts recommend taking it this way.

3. Incorporating It Into Your Diet:

You don't have to take it as a medicine. Instead, you can incorporate it into your diet, ensuring you consume the recommended amount - 15ml or one tablespoon - spread across your meals throughout the day.

The easiest way to do this is by using ACV as a salad dressing. It's perfectly fine to mix it with extra virgin olive oil. You can also add it to veggies or any other dishes you think it pairs well with, as long as it's not cooked.

You don't need to use the entire amount at once - you can spread it across multiple meals, such as two salads: one for lunch and one for dinner, for example.

This is how I used ACV. After my diagnosis, I didn't know about taking it as a morning supplement, but I did incorporate it into my diet and consumed it (almost) daily. I have since reversed my fatty liver, so I believe it definitely helped!

Are there any side effects to taking ACV?

First of all, it's important to note that ACV generally has no side effects. Some studies have linked it to potential damage to teeth due to its acidic nature, but this is typically prevented by diluting it in water.

There are also studies that suggest ACV could lead to reduced potassium levels or similar issues, but these cases are rare and usually involve people consuming very large amounts of undiluted apple cider vinegar (over 200ml per day), sometimes for years. So, from this perspective, we can consider it a very safe product when used daily in moderation (no more than 30ml or two tablespoons per day).

There are other potential issues, such as heartburn or its unpleasant taste, but these side effects are typically mitigated by following the recommended methods in steps #2 and especially #3 from the previous section.

Additionally, ACV may interact with certain medications, particularly diabetes medications. People who take both diabetes medication and ACV could experience dangerously low blood sugar or potassium levels. If you're on diabetes medication, be sure to consult your doctor before starting ACV.

For how long should you take apple cider vinegar?

Although some consider it a miracle cure, that's not the case. Apple Cider Vinegar is highly beneficial and can help with weight and fat loss, which contributes to reversing

NAFLD/MASLD, but it won't work overnight and won't be effective without accompanying lifestyle changes and improvements to your diet.

You should take ACV for at least 30 days. I recommend transitioning from taking it as a morning supplement (which shouldn't be done for too long - probably just the first 30 days) to incorporating it as a regular part of your diet.

Use the recommended amount (1-2 tablespoons) daily or as often as possible, such as in homemade salad dressings or to enhance the flavor of your meals. This way, you can take it naturally and enjoy its benefits for life.

4.3 The Liver-Friendly Superfoods

Regularly consuming the liver-friendly superfoods listed below will help you reverse your fatty liver faster and maintain your liver's health in the long term, as long as you combine them with my modified Mediterranean diet or any other healthy diet for NAFLD. As with all foods related to fatty liver, moderation is key. So don't go overboard and eat them in excessive amounts!

A word of caution before we dive into these liver-cleansing foods:

While these foods are excellent for your liver and have been proven - through both traditional use and scientific research in some cases - to have a beneficial effect, they are not a miracle cure on their own.

You will still need to follow a healthy, balanced diet recommended for fatty liver disease. You will still need to exercise and avoid the foods you shouldn't be eating. In other words, you still have to put in the effort.

In other words, you can't eat a pound of French fries with

deep-fried chicken wings every day and then consume these liver-cleansing superfoods, saying that you're doing your best. But incorporating these liver-friendly superfoods will definitely help give your liver a chance to recover faster.

You don't need to eat all of these foods every day, and you can also skip the ones you don't particularly enjoy. However, if you can include them all, that's even better. Consuming them regularly will provide your liver with the vitamins, minerals, and antioxidants it needs. Let's take a look at them!

Beetroot/Beets

I consider beetroot to be the ultimate superfood for liver cleansing - a must-eat, no matter what (so even if you don't like the taste). You should eat beets as often as possible. It's that good for the liver!

Beetroots are packed with minerals, vitamins, and antioxidants. They are rich in iron, calcium, Vitamin C, B vitamins, potassium, and dietary fiber. One of the fibers, pectin, is believed to stimulate the cleansing and removal of toxins from the liver.

Garlic

Sure, it might not smell great, but it's incredibly healthy - and not just for the liver.

When it comes to supporting liver health, garlic is believed to activate liver enzymes, helping the liver filter out toxins more efficiently. It's also known for reducing cholesterol and triglyceride levels.

For the best results, consume garlic raw, as cooking destroys many of its beneficial components. The good news is you don't need large amounts: two cloves a day should be enough to give your body the boost it needs to keep your liver healthy and speed up the reversal of NAFLD/MASLD.

Grapefruit

While all citrus fruits are considered beneficial for the liver, grapefruit stands out due to its high levels of vitamin C, antioxidants, and the liver-cleansing compound glutathione.

However, if you are on any medications, be sure to consult

your doctor before consuming grapefruit, as it can interact with various medications.

Turmeric (aka Curcuma)

Many consider turmeric the liver's favorite spice, as it's thought to provide more liver benefits than any other spice.

Despite its strong color, turmeric has a mild flavor, so you can easily add it to most dishes without significantly altering their taste.

Turmeric, with its high glutathione contents, is believed to help regenerate damaged liver cells and the overall liver detoxification process. Make this your go-to spice from now on!

Spinach

Popeye's favorite food should be yours too - and not just because of its relatively high iron content.

Spinach, like all leafy greens, helps neutralize heavy metals and pesticides, allowing your liver to flush out these harmful chemicals more effectively. Spinach also contains the enzyme glutathione, a key ally for your liver.

Extra Virgin Olive Oil (EVOO)

When it comes to reversing fatty liver, there's only one type of oil you should use: extra virgin olive oil. I've mentioned it multiple times throughout this book, but it's important to include it on this list because it's truly that good!

Offering a perfect combination of antioxidants and unsaturated fats, olive oil is great for your liver when consumed in moderation as part of a balanced, fatty liver-friendly diet, like the one I've recommended.

Use minimal quantities, though, and try to consume it raw to preserve its beneficial properties (so avoid cooking with it).

Avocado

This fat-rich fruit has become my favorite since being diagnosed with fatty liver. It's packed with glutathione, along with plenty other vitamins and minerals.

The high content of monounsaturated fat (the healthy kind) helps reduce bad cholesterol. Additionally, studies suggest that avocado supports liver detoxification and may even help reduce liver damage. The best part? It's delicious!

Walnuts

Walnuts are one of the few natural sources of arginine, an amino acid believed to greatly benefit the liver. They are also high in omega-3 fatty acids (similar to those found in fish) and contain glutathione.

Just be careful not to overeat, as walnuts pack a pretty high caloric punch!

4.4 Weight Loss Drugs: My Opinion

Even though there is still no medicine directly aimed at treating fatty liver disease, there has been some progress in this field, and we now have medications like Rezdiffra, which has been approved by the U.S. Food and Drug Administration for use in NASH (also known as MASH) patients with moderate to advanced liver scarring (fibrosis).

There are also some other, more controversial options, like Ozempic and Wegovy, which some fatty liver disease patients use to lose weight. However, these drugs are not specifically intended for reversing fatty liver disease, and they are relatively new to the market, so more studies are needed to fully understand their potential side effects.

Ozempic is FDA-approved for Type 2 diabetes and for lowering cardiovascular risk in certain patients (unrelated to fatty liver disease), while Wegovy is FDA-approved for weight loss and for reducing the risk of major cardiovascular events in overweight or obese adults.

Despite these differences in approval, both medications contain the same active ingredient: semaglutide. This is a glucagon-like peptide-1 (GLP-1) receptor agonist, which works by slowing digestion and reducing appetite, thus being believed to help with weight loss.

While there are many success stories you can read if you do some research, I know of one person who took Ozempic and didn't lose any weight (they didn't make any other changes to support weight loss, though). So, no, I don't believe this is the miracle cure that people with fatty liver disease are hoping for. Not only are these medications (which are actually injections) not directly targeted at treating fatty liver disease (MASH), but they may not work for everyone.

Nothing beats a proper diet and exercise when it comes to reversing fatty liver disease. However, if a trusted doctor prescribes these or any medication, it's important to follow their advice.

As for Rezdiffra, this is the one to watch, as it is at least aimed at helping people with liver disease. While it is not intended for fatty liver disease patients specifically - at least not at the moment of writing this book - it is for those with NASH (non-alcoholic steatohepatitis), which is a more advanced form of fatty liver disease.

Rezdiffra is a partial activator of a thyroid hormone receptor, which helps reduce liver fat accumulation. The results are promising: up to 36% of patients taking this drug experienced NASH resolution with no worsening of liver scarring, compared to a maximum of 13% in those who received only placebo and counseling on diet and exercise.

However, Rezdiffra is even newer than Ozempic and Wegovy, very expensive for most patients, and not intended for those with "just" fatty liver disease.

In conclusion, I believe we're still some time away from having a pill that can reverse fatty liver disease. And relying on a pill may not be the best approach. Fatty liver disease usually develops as a result of poor lifestyle choices, like unhealthy eating and lack of physical activity. Taking a pill won't change those habits, and if we continue to live unhealthily, the long-term effects on our overall health will be serious.

Therefore, unless a professional prescribes any type of medication, don't take it based on rumors or isolated cases. Instead, focus on healthy eating and regular exercise, and you will naturally reverse your condition, as so many others have, including myself.

5. Juicing and Fatty Liver

Juicing refers to making fresh juices at home from fruits, vegetables or a mixture of the two. Some people claim that the vitamins and minerals from juices are absorbed better than from whole fruits. However, this is generally not true.

In fact, when you juice fruits and vegetables, you lose most nutrients, including some vitamins and minerals, but especially fiber, which is essential for digestion.

This means that even freshly-squeezed juices can be more harmful than you'd believe them to be due to their high sugar content. The sugar in the juice is absorbed more quickly by the body because the fiber, which slows sugar absorption, is removed along with the pulp.

There are many "detox" diets and fruit/vegetable juice combinations that are said to cleanse the body, remove toxins, and help reverse fatty liver disease faster. Unfortunately, there is no scientific evidence to support these claims.

While it's true that drinking freshly squeezed juice is

better than not consuming fruits and vegetables at all, and that it gives your digestive system a break from dealing with fiber (which is a problem only for a very small number of people), it is by no means better than eating the whole fruit or vegetable.

A better alternative is preparing smoothies. Unlike juices, smoothies retain all the fiber and nutrients from the ingredients. They also taste great and can help you incorporate healthy foods you might not normally eat on their own.

So, if you want a more liquid form of fruits and vegetables, opt for smoothies instead of juices.

When making smoothies, try to use 70-80% vegetables and 30-20% fruits. Mix and match ingredients to include as many liver-friendly superfoods and other healthy options as possible. Only prepare enough for one meal or snack, and avoid adding sugar, honey, or flavor enhancers. Stick to just fruits, vegetables, and water if needed. Extra nuts and seeds - and even a bit of oil is permitted if you really feel the need to add these.

While I'm not personally a fan of smoothies, as I don't

enjoy the texture and prefer eating whole fruits and vegetables instead, I can recommend two recipes for liver-friendly smoothies. They make a great snack or breakfast.

For both recipes, wash and clean the ingredients, cut them into pieces, and blend them together (adding extra water if necessary). Consume them immediately.

1. Green smoothie

- 1 green apple, cored and chopped
- 1 cucumber, chopped
- 2 celery stalks, chopped
- 1 handful of kale
- 1 handful of spinach
- Half a lemon (peeled and deseeded)
- Half a cup parsley (chopped)
- 1/2 cup water (or less/more, as needed)

2. Beetroot & Carrot smoothie

- 1 small beetroot, peeled and chopped

- 1 small carrot, peeled and chopped

- 1 small green apple (or half of a regular one), cored and chopped

- 1 lemon (peeled and deseeded)

- 1-inch piece of ginger, grated

- 1/2 cup water

6. Intermittent Fasting and Fatty Liver

Intermittent fasting has gained increasing popularity recently, and its benefits appear to be supported by scientific evidence, which is always nice to see. Considered to be a healthy approach to living our lives, intermittent fasting seems to be effective in reducing fat in the liver and improving overall liver function, which is essential for reversing fatty liver disease.

For instance, a study from the *Egyptian Liver Journal* found that a regular diet combined with alternate-day fasting can actually reverse grade-1 fatty liver disease, now known as MASLD.

Additionally, Magnus Homler, MD, and his colleagues from the Department of Medicine at the Karolinska Institute in Stockholm, Sweden, found that a 5:2 diet, combined with a low-carb, high-fat approach, is very effective in reducing both body weight and hepatic steatosis (fatty liver).

Fasting increases the activity of certain enzymes that help break down fats. It also reduces liver inflammation. During fasting, pro-inflammatory markers, blood pressure, body weight, and fat levels are lower than usual. As a result, there is general agreement among health experts that fasting is indeed beneficial.

The best part is that I haven't come across any studies suggesting that fasting wouldn't benefit someone with fatty liver disease. This is promising news, but before making any major changes, be sure to consult your doctor!

While experts agree that fasting is generally healthy, some health conditions (such as diabetes) may make fasting risky or unsuitable. Also, it's important to note that fasting is not required to reverse fatty liver disease. It is one of the newer approaches that appears to help, but I personally did not practice intermittent fasting and was still able to reverse my fatty liver.

This doesn't mean I'm against intermittent fasting or that I believe it's ineffective. I just want to emphasize that if you find fasting very difficult (I do, for example), you can still get healthy by following a proper diet, exercising, and making my recommended lifestyle changes.

How Often Should You Fast if You Have a Fatty Liver?

There are three common methods of fasting:

1. **Daily time-restricted feeding** – also known as the "16:8 approach." You fast for 16 hours and eat your meals within an 8-hour window each day.

2. **Periodic fasting** – also called the "5:2 diet." You eat normally for 5 days a week and restrict your calorie intake on the other 2 days.

3. **Alternate-day fasting** – as the name suggests, you fast every other day.

Which method you choose depends on your personal preference, but I must say this again - do not start any fasting regimen without consulting your doctor first!

It's also important to maintain healthy eating habits while fasting. For example, if you only eat during a 2-hour window each day but consume 5,000 calories of unhealthy food, you will most likely still gain weight and not experience any benefits from fasting.

What Can I Eat While Fasting?

During your fasting periods, you can drink water and zero-calorie beverages, such as unsweetened tea and black coffee, but nothing else.

During your eating periods, you can eat normally. By "normal," I mean following a healthy and nutritious diet, like the Mediterranean diet I recommended in this book. It's crucial to avoid high-calorie junk food, fried foods, and sugary treats, as these are harmful to the liver and overall health.

In other words, starting intermittent fasting doesn't mean you can ignore what or how much you eat during your eating windows, nor that you are free not to follow a proper diet that.

While there are still many questions to be answered about the relationship between intermittent fasting and fatty liver, the current evidence is promising. However, if fasting feels too extreme or difficult, it's not mandatory. You can still reverse fatty liver by eating healthy meals each day, exercising, and taking care of your overall well-being.

7. Fatty Liver-Friendly Recipes & Meal Plan

The question I get asked most often - and the one I asked myself repeatedly after being diagnosed with fatty liver disease - is: **What do I eat?**

Understanding the basic principles (what we did until now) is helpful, but many of us struggle when it comes to putting those principles into practice and creating healthy meals from scratch. Trust me: it gets easier the more you do it. To help you get started, I will share a variety of recipes you can try before you begin making your own.

I hope you find these recipes as helpful as I want them to be. I've organized them by the time of day you might eat them, but don't feel restricted by this. You can have something listed for breakfast at lunch or dinner, and vice versa. I'll also provide a recommended meal plan for a week - something to help you get started on the right foot while keeping your diet as varied as possible.

There are countless other options out there, but hopefully

these will give you a great starting point and solid ideas for meals while you work on reversing your fatty liver.

7.1 Breakfast Ideas & Recipes

Note: Except for the first recipe below, all portions are for one serving.

Homemade Hummus

Ingredients:

- 1 cup chickpeas (soak overnight in 4 cups of water)

- 4 tablespoons organic tahini

- 2 garlic cloves

- Juice from half a lemon

- ½ teaspoon each of pepper flakes or paprika and ground cumin

- Salt to taste

Instructions:

1. Rinse the chickpeas after soaking and transfer them to a large pot, covering them with about 8 cups of water. Bring to a boil, reduce heat to low, and simmer for around 50 minutes.

2. Once done, drain the chickpeas, but keep 1–2 cups

of the cooking water. Transfer the chickpeas to a food processor.

3. In the processor, add garlic cloves, lemon juice, tahini, paprika, cumin, and salt. Add ½ cup of the reserved cooking water. Puree until creamy.

Note: Adjust creaminess by adding more water if necessary. I usually end up adding around 1 cup. Experiment to find the consistency you prefer.

Optional: You can add baked red peppers to the mix for extra color and flavor. For the ingredients above, one paprika will do the trick.

4. Transfer the hummus to a bowl and enjoy. You can sprinkle extra paprika on top, but avoid adding extra oil - tahini already contains enough fat and calories.

You can enjoy the hummus on its own, spread on whole wheat bread (preferably homemade), or with vegetables such as cucumber, zucchini, salad greens, or kale. It also works as a dipping sauce for falafel or with healthy tortilla chips.

Chia Seeds Pudding

Ingredients:

- 3 tablespoons chia seeds
- 10 tablespoons water (or 50% water, 50% low-fat milk)
- ½ teaspoon honey
- ¼ cup fresh berries (I prefer blueberries and raspberries, but any berries work!)
- 1 teaspoon coconut flakes
- ¼ teaspoon Ceylon cinnamon (this is the best type of cinnamon to use)
- 1 teaspoon roasted almond flakes (or other nuts/seeds)

Instructions:

1. In a bowl, mix water (or the water/milk combination), chia seeds, and honey. Let the mixture sit for 10 minutes.

2. Stir again, then add the remaining ingredients in stages: start with the coconut flakes, stir well, then add the almond flakes, stir again, and add the cinnamon (stir once more). Finally, top with the berries.

3. Let it sit for 5 more minutes, give it a final stir, and enjoy your delicious, fatty liver-friendly chia pudding!

—

Oats (Porridge)

Ingredients:

- 4 tablespoons oat flakes (steel-cut are ideal, but rolled oats work too)

- ½ cup water

- ½ cup low-fat milk (for a lighter option, use just water; for a richer taste, use more milk. I prefer a balance of both)

- ¼ cup frozen or fresh blueberries

- 2 tablespoons raspberries

- ⅓ of a medium banana, sliced

- 1 teaspoon coconut flakes

- ¼ teaspoon Ceylon cinnamon

Instructions:

1. Heat the milk and water in a pot over medium heat. After a couple of minutes, add the oat flakes and stir continuously.

2. When the mixture starts to boil, reduce the heat to low and let it simmer for 3 more minutes, continuing to stir.

3. Add the fruits and stir for another minute. Once cooked, transfer the mixture to a bowl, top with coconut flakes and cinnamon, and enjoy.

Overnight Oats Variation: If you prefer not to boil the oats, you can prepare overnight oats (which I've recently switched to). Simply place the oats in a bowl with the milk and water mixture and let them sit overnight. In the morning, add the fruits (fresh or frozen) and microwave for 1 minute (or longer if you prefer it warmer). Add the cinnamon and coconut flakes at the end, and enjoy your faster, no-boil breakfast!

Note: I listed the fruits I use, but feel free to substitute with any fresh or frozen fruits in different proportions. Customize it with the fruits you enjoy, although I think you'll love my version!

—

Yogurt and Berries

Ingredients:

- 120 grams (about ½ cup) low-fat yogurt (1% to max 3.5% fat)
- 2 tablespoons berries of your choice
- Optional: sprinkle some peanuts, walnuts, or pistachios on top

Simply mix all the ingredients together and eat them fresh.

—

Toast with Avocado and Ricotta

Ingredients:

- ½ avocado, peeled and sliced

- 1 tablespoon ricotta cheese

- 1 slice whole wheat bread, toasted

- Salt and pepper to taste

- Optional: 1 clove garlic and/or paprika flakes

- Optional: 1 slice of tomato

Spread the ricotta cheese over the toast and place the avocado slices on top. Season with paprika flakes, salt, and pepper (or skip the spices if preferred).

For extra flavor, rub a garlic clove over the warm toast before adding the avocado and ricotta. You can also add a slice of tomato for more taste and nutrition.

—

Skinny Omelet

Ingredients:

- 1 medium-sized whole egg, beaten

- Egg whites from 1 medium-sized egg, beaten

- A few feta cheese cubes (max 50 grams/0.11 lbs)

- 1 spring onion, chopped

- A handful of arugula (rucola) leaves

- ½ tomato

- Salt and pepper to taste

Mix the beaten egg and egg whites with a bit of salt and pepper, then pour the mixture into a non-stick skillet heated over medium heat for a couple of minutes. Tilt the skillet so the egg mixture spreads evenly across the surface.

Let the eggs cook until the bottom is partially set (usually 30-60 seconds), then use a spatula to flip it over.

While the other side is cooking, add the crumbled feta cheese and chopped onion. Let it cook for about 1 more minute, then remove the skillet from the heat. Add the arugula leaves and carefully roll the omelet.

Transfer to a plate, cut the half tomato into pieces, and enjoy!

7.2 Lunch Ideas & Recipes

Minestrone Soup

Ingredients:

- 2 large red onions, chopped
- 2 cloves garlic, minced
- 2 cups chopped celery
- 3 large carrots, diced
- 1 cup green beans, cut into ½-inch pieces
- 1.5 cups dried kidney beans
- 1 large bell pepper, diced
- 1 cup frozen peas
- 1 can diced tomatoes
- 2 cups tomato sauce (100% tomato content)
- 2 tablespoons fresh basil (or 1 teaspoon dried basil)
- 6 cups water
- Salt to taste
- 1 tablespoon grated Parmesan cheese for topping (optional)

Instructions:

1. Add the onions, carrots, and celery to a large stock pot and bring to a boil over medium heat in the 6 cups of water.

2. Once boiling, add the green beans, bell pepper, frozen peas, and diced tomatoes. Continue boiling for an additional 30 minutes. Add more water if necessary—it should be thick, like a stew.

3. After 30 minutes, add the tomato sauce, basil, and salt to taste. Let it simmer for 5–10 more minutes, then add the garlic and let it simmer for another 5 minutes (or longer if the vegetables are not fully cooked).

4. When serving, sprinkle Parmesan over the minestrone soup. It's absolutely delicious!

—

Vegetable Soup

Ingredients:

- 1 kg/2 lbs baby carrots (frozen is fine)

- 2 peeled onions (whole)
- Root of 1 medium celery
- 2 medium potatoes, cubed
- 2.5 liters (85 oz) water
- 1 teaspoon turmeric powder
- Salt & pepper to taste
- Fresh parsley for topping

Instructions:

1. Place the frozen baby carrots, celery root, and whole onions in a pot of water and boil over medium heat for 20 minutes.

2. Add the cubed potatoes, turmeric powder, salt, and pepper. Stir and continue boiling for another 20 minutes, until the potatoes are thoroughly cooked. Add more water if needed.

3. When ready, remove the onions and celery root (you can chop these and mix with peas, grated apples, and carrots for a tasty salad). Serve the soup warm, topped

with freshly cut parsley. Enjoy this healthy, low-calorie soup daily!

—

Chicken Hummus Bowl

Ingredients:

- 1 pound boneless, skinless chicken breast, cut into 1-inch pieces
- 2 cups homemade hummus (use the recipe from this book)
- 2 tablespoons extra virgin olive oil (EVOO)
- 1 teaspoon each of paprika and ground cumin
- 14 oz cherry tomatoes, halved
- 1 large cucumber, sliced
- 1 red onion, thinly sliced
- Fresh parsley to taste (about ¼ cup)
- 2 cloves garlic, mashed
- 2 tablespoons lemon juice
- Salt and pepper to taste (a pinch of each)

Instructions:

1. Mix the chicken breast pieces with 1 tablespoon of EVOO, paprika, cumin, salt, and pepper.

2. Preheat your oven to broil at 450°F. Place the chicken on a foil-lined baking sheet and broil in the upper third of the oven until cooked through, about 10 minutes.

3. While the chicken is cooking, mix the mashed garlic with a pinch of salt, lemon juice, and the remaining 1 tablespoon of EVOO.

4. Once the chicken is out of the oven, toss it in the garlic-lemon mixture and let it sit for 5–6 minutes.

5. Divide the hummus into 4 portions, using shallow bowls or plates. Top with the tomatoes, cucumber, onion, parsley, and chicken. Enjoy!

—

Healthy Chicken Shawarma

Ingredients:

- 1.1 lbs (500g) skinless, boneless chicken breast

- 1 tbsp each of ground cumin, turmeric powder, paprika, ground coriander, and garlic powder

- Cayenne pepper and salt to taste (around ½ teaspoon each)

- 1 tablespoon extra virgin olive oil (EVOO)

- ½ cup natural lemon juice

- 1 large red onion, thinly sliced

- 1 cup chopped cabbage

- 1 cup cherry tomatoes, halved

- 1 cucumber, sliced

- 1 large red pepper, chopped

- **Sauce:** 1 cup low-fat yogurt (1.5% fat, no sugar) and 1 garlic clove, minced

- **To serve:** 4 whole wheat pita pockets (or ideally, replace them with salad leaves)

Instructions:

1. In a bowl, mix the cumin, turmeric, paprika, coriander, garlic powder, salt, and cayenne pepper. Set

aside.

2. Slice the chicken breast into bite-sized pieces and coat well with the spice mix. Add the oil and lemon juice, then cover the bowl and refrigerate for 3–12 hours (optional, but marinating improves flavor).

3. Preheat the oven to 425°F. Spread the chicken on a baking sheet and roast for 30 minutes, turning it over after 20 minutes (cook longer if you prefer the chicken crispier, but keep an eye on it).

4. When ready, divide the chicken into four portions. Prepare the pita pockets (or salad leaves) by spreading the yogurt and minced garlic mixture. Add the cabbage and vegetables (cucumber, red pepper, cherry tomatoes, and onion). Fill the pita pockets/leaves with the chicken, roll them up, and serve immediately.

—

Slow-Cooked Chicken Chili

Ingredients:

- 1.1 lbs (500g) skinless, boneless chicken breast

- 1 cup diced tomatoes

- ½ cup pinto beans (cooked or canned)

- ½ cup black beans (cooked or canned)

- 2 avocados, cut into bite-sized pieces

- 1 cup red cabbage (or any type of cabbage)

- Salt, pepper, and garlic powder to taste (around ⅓ teaspoon each)

- **Optional:** 4 tablespoons light sour cream and ¼ cup shredded light cheese

Note: To make it even healthier, you can skip the cheese and sour cream (or ideally, both).

Instructions:

1. Cut the chicken into bite-sized pieces and bake in a preheated oven at 425°F for 30 minutes (without oil or spices).

2. While the chicken is cooking, mix the tomatoes and beans, then season with salt and pepper.

3. Mix the cabbage with garlic powder and either combine with the beans or keep it as a topping.

4. Once the chicken is done, let it rest for 5 minutes, then mix with the beans and cabbage. Top with avocado, a tablespoon of light sour cream, and a sprinkle of cheese (optional).

—

Greek Salad

Ingredients:

- 1 large tomato, cut into bite-sized pieces
- 1 medium cucumber, sliced
- ½ red onion, chopped
- ½ bell pepper, sliced
- 5 Kalamata olives
- 1.4 oz (40g) Feta cheese or any white cheese
- 1 tablespoon EVOO
- ½ teaspoon oregano
- Salt and ground pepper to taste

Instructions:

Mix all the ingredients together and enjoy your salad fresh!

—

Lentil Stew with Poached Egg

Ingredients:

- ½ cup cooked red lentils
- ¾ cup fresh baby spinach & arugula leaves
- 1 small tomato, chopped
- 1 poached egg

Instructions: Mix everything together into a delicious, albeit messy-looking, meal. Sometimes the best-tasting dishes aren't the prettiest!

—

Eggplant Boats

Ingredients:

- 1 eggplant, cut in half
- 3 tablespoons water

- 2 medium red onions, chopped

- 1 red pepper, finely chopped

- ½ cup 100% tomato juice or minced tomatoes

- 2.8 oz (80 grams) low-fat cheese, grated

- Green onions or parsley for topping

- Salt & ground pepper to taste (optional: paprika or chili flakes for extra spice)

Instructions:

1. Preheat the oven to 350°F. Place the eggplant halves on a tray and bake for about 30 minutes.

2. While the eggplant is baking, sauté the onions in water for about 3 minutes, then add the red pepper and cook for another 3 minutes. Add more water if necessary. Finally, add the tomato juice and let everything simmer for 5-7 minutes.

3. Once the eggplants are cooked, scoop out the flesh, leaving the skins intact.

4. Mix the scooped eggplant with the onion and

197

pepper mixture. Add spices to taste, then spoon the mixture back into the eggplant shells. Sprinkle grated cheese on top.

5. Return the eggplants to the oven at 400°F for 10 more minutes, or until the cheese is crispy.

6. Garnish with green onions or parsley and enjoy straight from the eggplant shells while warm.

—

Grilled Chicken Breast with Green Leaves Salad

Ingredients:

- 7 oz (200 grams) chicken breast fillet, boneless and skinless
- Salt & pepper to taste
- 1 spring onion, chopped, for topping
- ¼ cup fresh beetroot, grated
- ¼ cup carrots, grated
- ½ cup baby spinach
- 1 teaspoon extra virgin olive oil (EVOO)

- 1 tablespoon apple cider vinegar (ACV)

Instructions:

1. Grill the chicken breast until cooked through, then season with salt and pepper. Top with chopped spring onion.

2. Mix the grated vegetables and spinach with EVOO and ACV. Serve as a side dish with the chicken. Fast, easy, and healthy!

Note: You can substitute any salad, such as the Greek salad mentioned earlier or a simple green salad with spinach, lettuce, arugula, and spring onions, dressed with EVOO and ACV.

—

Low-Fat Tuna Wrap

Ingredients:

- 6 oz tuna (canned, in water)
- 1 whole-wheat wrap
- 2 teaspoons low-fat yogurt
- ¼ red onion, chopped

- ½ celery stalk, chopped

- A handful of raw baby spinach leaves

- Juice from ½ lemon

- Optional: a sprinkle of chili flakes (for added spice)

Instructions:

1. Drain the tuna and mix it with lemon juice. Sprinkle chili flakes if using.

2. Spread the yogurt evenly on the whole-wheat wrap and top with the tuna.

3. Add the spinach leaves, chopped onion, and celery. Roll the wrap and enjoy!

—

Quinoa Salad with Beans

Ingredients:

- ½ cup cooked quinoa

- ¼ cup black beans, rinsed and drained

- ¼ cup corn kernels

- 1 red bell pepper, diced

- ½ onion, chopped

- ¼ cup cherry tomatoes, halved (optional)

- ¼ cup fresh cilantro, chopped (optional)

- Juice from ½ lime

- Salt and pepper to taste

- ½ teaspoon ground cumin

- ½ teaspoon paprika

Instructions:

1. In a large bowl, combine the cooked quinoa, black beans, corn, diced red bell pepper, and chopped onion. Add cherry tomatoes and cilantro if desired.

2. Squeeze the lime juice over the mixture. Season with salt, pepper, cumin, and paprika.

3. Toss everything together until well combined. Serve immediately, or let it sit in the refrigerator for 30 minutes to allow the flavors to meld.

7.3 Dinner Ideas & Recipes

Garlic Salmon with Vegetables

Ingredients:

- 21 oz (600 grams) wild salmon fillet

- 1 teaspoon each of parsley and garlic powder

- Salt and black pepper to taste

- Juice from ½ to 1 whole lemon

- Vegetable salad of choice (greens work best: lettuce, arugula, baby spinach, cucumber, and cherry tomatoes)

Instructions:

1. Place the salmon on a baking sheet in a baking tray. Mix the parsley, garlic powder, salt, and lemon juice, then brush the mixture over the salmon. (If there isn't enough liquid, add a little water.)

2. Preheat the oven to 400°F (200°C). Cover the tray with a lid or aluminum foil. Bake for around 25 minutes, or until the salmon is cooked to your liking. (For a crispier finish, remove the cover after 15 minutes.)

3. Serve the salmon with a side of vegetables and top with freshly squeezed lemon juice.

—

Healthy Tuna Salad

Ingredients:

- 1 can tuna chunks in water (drained weight: 4 oz / 110g)
- 1 cup lettuce, chopped
- 1 small red onion (or ½ a medium onion), chopped
- 4 cherry tomatoes, halved
- 5 Kalamata olives (or any olives you prefer)
- 1 teaspoon extra virgin olive oil (EVOO)
- 2 teaspoons fresh lemon juice
- ½ teaspoon dried oregano
- 1 teaspoon apple cider vinegar (optional)
- Salt and ground black pepper to taste

Instructions:

1. Drain the water from the tuna and transfer it to a

bowl.

2. Add all the remaining ingredients and mix well. Serve immediately.

—

Beans & Chickpea Salad

Ingredients:

- 15 oz each of black beans, chickpeas, and kidney beans (rinsed in cold water)
- 1 medium red onion, chopped
- 2 stalks of celery, chopped
- 2 cloves garlic, minced
- ½ teaspoon cumin, salt, and chopped parsley (adjust to taste; you can use more parsley)
- 2 tablespoons extra virgin olive oil
- 1 tablespoon apple cider vinegar (ACV)

Instructions:

1. Mix all the ingredients in a large bowl.

2. Refrigerate for at least an hour before serving to let

the flavors meld. Enjoy this simple and delicious dish!

—

Three Beans Salad (Mediterranean Style)

Note: This recipe is very similar to the Beans & Chickpea Salad I shared earlier. Personally, I prefer this version because I don't enjoy the taste of chickpeas in anything but hummus. If you feel the same, this salad will be perfect for you too!

Ingredients:

- 1 can (15 oz) each of black beans, red beans, and white beans (drained and rinsed)
- 1 medium tomato, chopped
- ½ red pepper, chopped
- 1 small red onion, chopped
- 4 tablespoons sweet corn (no added sugar)
- Juice from ½ a lemon OR 2 tablespoons apple cider vinegar
- 1 tablespoon extra virgin olive oil (EVOO)
- 1 teaspoon mustard

- **Optional:** 1 stalk of celery, chopped (for extra crunch)

Instructions:

Simply mix all the ingredients in a large bowl and let it sit in the fridge for 1 hour before serving. It's really easy to prepare and delicious!

—

Cauliflower Buffalo "Wings"

Ingredients:

- 1 bag (10 oz / 300g) cauliflower florets
- ½ teaspoon each of paprika, garlic powder, and onion powder
- 2 tablespoons Buffalo sauce
- Salt to taste
- **Optional dressing:** 1 cup low-fat yogurt (4 oz / 120g), 1 clove minced garlic, ½ tablespoon each of fresh parsley and dill

Instructions:

1. Mix the paprika, garlic powder, onion powder, and a pinch of salt in a bowl.

2. Coat the cauliflower florets with the spice mix and roast them in a preheated oven at 400°F (200°C) for 15 minutes.

3. Increase the oven temperature to 450°F (230°C). Move the cauliflower to a bowl, mix it with the Buffalo sauce, then return it to the oven for 5 more minutes.

4. Serve warm as is, or use the optional dressing by mixing the yogurt with the other ingredients for a tasty dipping sauce.

—

Zucchini Roll-ups

Ingredients:

- 2 medium zucchini
- 2 red onions, diced
- 2 sweet peppers, diced
- 1 cup carrots, shredded

- ½ cup baby spinach

- 1 can diced tomatoes (14 oz / 400g)

- 2 cloves garlic, minced

- Salt and pepper to taste (usually around ¼ teaspoon)

- **Optional:** ¼ cup parmesan

Instructions:

1. Sauté all the vegetables except for the zucchini in ¼ cup of water (no oil necessary). You can puree the tomatoes if you prefer a thicker consistency. Add the minced garlic 2 minutes before stopping the cooking. Stir regularly.

2. While the vegetables are cooking, wash the zucchini and use a peeler to create flat, wide slices for rolling.

3. Layer 3 slices of zucchini to form a larger roll, then top with the sautéed vegetables. Roll them up and place them on a baking sheet. Pour any leftover juice over the rolls.

4. Bake in a preheated oven at 400°F for 15 minutes.

When ready, serve warm or sprinkle with parmesan or any grated cheese, if desired.

—

Hearty Carrot & Beet Salad

Ingredients:

- 2 large carrots, grated
- 1 medium-sized beet, grated
- 1 teaspoon EVOO
- 1 tablespoon apple cider vinegar
- Salt and pepper to taste

Instructions:

Mix all the ingredients together. You can enjoy this salad as your main dish for lunch, or serve half of it as a side with your main course, such as grilled chicken breast or the garlic salmon from earlier in the book.

—

Grilled Chicken Fajita

This recipe might seem a bit more involved, but it's well

worth the effort! It's a healthier take on the classic fajita, with liver-friendly tweaks that the whole family will enjoy.

Ingredients (for 4 servings):

For the chicken:

- 4 chicken breast fillets (about 400 grams / 16 ounces)

- 1 red bell pepper (or half red and half yellow for more color)

- 1 medium onion, sliced

- 4 cups Romaine leaves

- 4 avocado halves, sliced

For the dressing:

- 2 tablespoons olive oil

- ¼ cup fresh lime juice (lemon works fine too)

- 2 cloves garlic, minced

- 2 tablespoons cilantro, chopped

- ½ teaspoon cumin

- 1 teaspoon red chili (or red pepper flakes if you

prefer less heat)

- 1 teaspoon salt

How to Prepare:

The Dressing: Mix all the dressing ingredients together before you start cooking the meat and set aside.

The Chicken:

1. Grill the chicken fillets in a non-stick pan (no oil needed) on both sides until cooked through. Set aside to rest.

2. In the same pan, add the sliced bell pepper and cook for about 2 minutes, adding a bit of water if needed. Set aside when done.

3. Slice the chicken fillets into strips and place over the Romaine leaves. Add the pepper slices, onion, and avocado, then drizzle with the dressing. Enjoy with your family!

—

Chicken Vegetable Skillet

211

Ingredients:

- ½ lb chicken breast, cut into strips

- 1 small onion, chopped

- ½ cup carrots, grated

- 1 zucchini, sliced

- ½ bell pepper, chopped

- 2 tablespoons water (if needed)

- Salt & pepper to taste

- 1 teaspoon garlic powder (optional)

Instructions:

1. Heat a skillet over medium heat. Add the chicken strips and cook, stirring occasionally, until browned and cooked through. Remove the chicken and keep warm.

2. In the same skillet, add the onion, carrots, zucchini, and bell pepper. Cook for about 10 minutes, stirring occasionally, until the vegetables are tender. Add water if necessary to prevent sticking.

3. Return the chicken to the skillet. Season with salt,

212

pepper, and garlic powder (if using). Stir to combine and cook for 2-3 more minutes. Serve immediately.

—

Spinach Quesadillas

Ingredients:

- 4 cups fresh spinach
- 4 green onions, chopped (or 1 regular onion, chopped)
- 1 large tomato, chopped
- Juice from ½ lemon or 1 lime
- 1 teaspoon ground cumin
- ½ teaspoon garlic powder
- Salt to taste (optional)
- 1 cup low-fat shredded cheese (your favorite variety)
- 4-6 whole wheat tortillas (with minimal ingredients)

Instructions:

1. Heat a skillet over medium heat. Add the spinach, green onions (or regular onion), tomato, lemon juice, cumin, garlic powder, and salt (if using). Cook until the spinach is wilted and the vegetables are tender, about 7-10 minutes.

2. Transfer the cooked spinach mixture to a bowl. Stir in the shredded cheese until well combined. (If you don't want the cheese to melt yet, let the mixture cool slightly.)

3. Assemble the quesadillas: place a tortilla on a flat surface, spread a portion of the spinach and cheese mixture on one half, then fold the other half over.

4. Heat a griddle or large skillet over medium heat. Cook the folded quesadilla for 2 minutes on each side, or until the tortilla is golden brown and the cheese is melted.

7.4 Snacks & Other Recipes

You can enjoy these between meals if you're craving a snack or even adapt them for breakfast or a lighter lunch/dinner. While the options below are simple, they are satisfying, but also fast & easy to prepare at home.

Plain Popcorn

Make your own popcorn with no added fat or flavorings. Simply pop the corn in a microwave or on the stovetop. Enjoy two handfuls as a healthy snack.

—

Fruits

Fruits are great for snacking and help curb sugar cravings. Mix and match your favorites, but be sure to eat them in moderation. Here are some examples of fruit portions I typically eat (each line represents one portion):

- 1 banana
- 1 large apple
- 2 oranges

- 1 cup blueberries, raspberries, or strawberries

- 3-4 apricots

- 2 peaches

- 2 pears

—

Vegetables

Though they can be a tougher snack to get used to, vegetables are an amazing option. Feel free to mix and match to your preference. Below are some examples of vegetable portions I recommend:

- 1-2 medium carrots (you can cut them into sticks if you like)

- 1-2 cucumbers

- 1 bell pepper, sliced

- 2 radishes

- 2 celery sticks

—

Vegetable Chips (Homemade)

If fresh vegetables aren't your thing, you can make your own chips at home using potatoes, sweet potatoes, beets, or carrots.

1. Slice your vegetable of choice into very thin pieces (a mandoline works well for this) and lay them flat on a microwave-safe plate. Make sure they don't overlap.

2. Microwave on high for 1–1.5 minutes. When done, flip the slices and microwave the other side for another 1–1.5 minutes.

3. Let them cool, and you'll have healthy, crispy homemade chips that are friendly for a fatty liver diet!

These snacks are easy to prepare and provide healthy alternatives to processed options.

—

Yogurt

Enjoy 120 grams (4.2 ounces) of plain, low-fat yogurt with no added sugar. You can mix in a couple of teaspoons of berries (blueberries and raspberries are my favorites) or pair it with a couple of whole-wheat, ideally homemade, crackers.

—

Nuts and Seeds

You have plenty of options here: nuts, peanuts, Cajun, pistachios, almonds, sunflower seeds, pumpkin seeds - anything goes. Feel free to mix and match as you like.

Two important points to remember:

1. Keep portions small (max 50 grams or 1.75 ounces per serving) because they are calorie-packed.

2. Choose roasted (or raw, if possible) options instead of fried, and avoid products with added oil, chemicals, additives, or artificial flavors.

—

Smoothies

I discussed smoothies in a previous chapter and shared two recipes. To make things easier, here they are again. For both, simply mix the ingredients and blend them well (add more water if needed) and enjoy immediately:

Green Smoothie

- 1 green apple, cored and chopped
- 1 cucumber, chopped
- 2 celery stalks, chopped
- 1 handful kale
- 1 handful spinach
- ½ lemon, peeled and deseeded
- ½ cup parsley, chopped
- 1 cup water (adjust as needed)

Beetroot & Carrot Smoothie

- 1 small beetroot, peeled and chopped
- 1 small carrot, peeled and chopped
- 1 small green apple (or half of a larger one), cored and chopped
- 1 lemon, peeled and deseeded
- 1-inch piece of ginger, grated
- 1 cup water

—

Apple Slices with Peanut Butter

Slice half an apple and add a bit of 100% peanut butter for a healthy and delicious snack.

—

Beef Jerky

Many beef jerky products are full of chemicals, added sugars, and - surprisingly - aren't even 100% beef (they may include pork or chicken). Be sure to research brands that offer real, clean beef jerky, and enjoy a small portion as a snack.

—

Rainbow Whole Fruit Popsicles

Ingredients:

- Popsicle molds (for freezing the fruit)
- 1 cup banana, sliced
- 2 kiwi
- 1 cup strawberries
- 1 cup blueberries
- 1 cup pineapple

Puree each fruit separately in a food processor. If a puree is too thick (usually banana and strawberries), add a bit of water or low-fat milk.

Carefully spoon each fruit puree into the bottom of your popsicle mold, leveling it before freezing until solid. Repeat the process with each fruit until the popsicle is fully assembled. The result is a beautiful, colorful, and delicious treat.

If you prefer a quicker option, puree all the fruits together and freeze for a tasty frozen fruit cocktail.

—

Date & Coconut Balls

Ingredients:

- 1 cup pitted Medjool dates
- 1 cup shredded coconut
- ¼ cup shredded coconut for coating
- ½ cup roasted almonds or roasted Cajun nuts
- ¼ cup milk

In a small pot, heat the milk and Medjool dates over

medium heat for 5-6 minutes until warm but not boiling.

Transfer the dates and milk to a food processor, add the shredded coconut, and process in short bursts until well combined.

Scoop small portions with a teaspoon and roll them into balls around a whole almond or Cajun nut. Once formed, roll each ball in additional coconut flakes.

A serving size is 2-4 balls.

7.5 Meal Plan for a Week

While the recipes above provide plenty of options to diversify your meals, there are countless other dishes you can prepare to ensure your diet remains enjoyable and varied.

However, even with recipes in hand, many people struggle with how to mix and match their meals. This meal plan is designed to help guide you through seven days, using both recipes from the previous chapters and a few new suggestions.

My fatty liver meal plan follows a few main principles: low fat, low sugar/carbs, smaller portions, and a focus on healthy eating based on the Mediterranean diet that I personally follow. However, it may NOT be suitable for individuals with diabetes or other medical conditions. Still, those who have tried it have reported great results and a better understanding of how to eat to support their recovery.

I've made an effort to keep the plan as varied as possible, though there's nothing wrong with repeating meals (like overnight oats for breakfast) for a few days in a row. For the sake of demonstrating how diverse your menu can be, I'll provide a range of different meal examples below.

You can follow this meal plan exactly, modify it to your liking, or use it as inspiration to create your own. There is plenty of variety to be had when managing a fatty liver!

MONDAY

- **Breakfast**: Homemade porridge / oatmeal with blueberries.

- **1st Snack**: Handful of nuts, raw or roasted.

- **Lunch**: Mediterranean Salad (no bread!)

- **2nd Snack**: One Banana.

- **Dinner**: Grilled Turkey breast with black rice or brown rice.

TUESDAY

- **Breakfast**: Homemade guacamole on toast (use

wholewheat bread).

- **1st Snack**: One apple.

- **Lunch**: Homemade vegetable soup and quinoa with beans salad.

- **2nd Snack**: One cup of low fat yogurt (optional: add one whole-wheat cracker OR blueberries/strawberries).

- **Dinner**: Barley-Stuffed Poblanos/Peppers.

WEDNESDAY

- **Breakfast**: Chia pudding with berries.

- **1st Snack**: A cup of homemade popcorn.

- **Lunch**: One Eggplant Boat.

- **2nd Snack**: Two small carrots.

- **Dinner**: Garlic salmon with vegetables.

THURSDAY

- **Breakfast**: Skinny omelet.

- **1st Snack**: 2 celery sticks.

- **Lunch**: Minestrone soup.

- **2nd Snack**: Beetroot & carrot smoothie.

- **Dinner**: Cauliflower Buffalo "wings".

FRIDAY

- **Breakfast**: One apple, sliced, with peanut butter.

- **1st Snack**: Handful of nuts and seeds.

- **Lunch**: Three beans salad.

- **2nd Snack**: Cucumber sticks.

- **Dinner**: Low-fat tuna wrap.

SATURDAY

- **Breakfast**: Homemade hummus.

- **1st Snack**: One cup of low fat yogurt and berries.

- **Lunch**: Lentil salad with poached eggs and beets salad.

- **2nd Snack**: Carrot sticks.

- **Dinner**: Chicken vegetable skillet.

SUNDAY

- **Breakfast**: Toast with ricotta and sundried tomatoes.

- **1st Snack**: Date & coconut balls.

- **Lunch**: Grilled chicken fajitas.

- **2nd Snack**: Green smoothie.

- **Dinner**: Spinach quesadillas.

8. Keeping Your Liver Healthy After Reversing Fatty Liver Disease

You've reversed your fatty liver! Time to pop a bottle of champagne, order cake, and party all night to celebrate, right?

Well... not so fast!

Even after reversing your fatty liver disease (which I'm confident you will do if you follow the advice in this book), it's essential to maintain your diet, continue exercising, and stick to the new lifestyle you've built.

The fatty liver diet isn't like a typical diet where you follow it for a week or a month and then return to old habits. If you do, as with any diet, you'll likely regain the weight (and often faster than you lost it), and your fatty liver will return. Yo-yoing between healthy and unhealthy habits puts additional stress on your body and liver, and reversing it a second time will be even more challenging.

Instead, you need to continue eating healthy, balanced

meals and staying active. The truth is, if you've managed to reverse fatty liver disease, you're already feeling much better than you did before. You feel more comfortable in your own skin, have more energy, sleep better, have a more positive mood, and generally enjoy life more.

This is the opposite of how you may have felt when you first started, when you thought you'd be missing out on all the delicious food and drinks you used to enjoy. You might have worried that life wouldn't be as fun anymore, but now you know that feeling healthy is far better, and no burger or sweet treat can give you that same sense of well-being.

So, make sure to stick to your new lifestyle—especially when it comes to eating and exercising—for the long term.

For example, I stopped drinking alcohol when I was diagnosed and haven't had a sip since. Not on my birthday, not on special occasions—never. And while I'm not always as strict about food as I was at the beginning (I occasionally allow myself a burger and fries, half a pizza, or a piece of cake, and even a

Snickers every now and then), I still generally stick to the Mediterranean diet, keep my weight under control, and eat much healthier and cleaner than I did before my NAFLD diagnosis.

If I can do it (and I've been doing it for over 10 years now), anyone can. And everyone should, especially after reversing fatty liver. You now know how beneficial healthy eating and staying active are, and how great it makes you feel. There's no reason to return to old habits just because that's how you used to be. In fact, that's exactly why you shouldn't—because the "old you" was likely overweight, low on energy, and generally unhealthy. Embrace and stick to being the new, healthier you!

Most importantly, always take a moment to look in the mirror and congratulate yourself on your achievement. Although it's relatively easy to reverse fatty liver if you stick to the plan, few people actually manage to do it. You're one of them. You're one of the winners. You're one of the doers.

Congratulations!

9. Closing words

Thank you for reading this book. Unlike many similar ones on the market, I wrote it based on my personal experience overcoming fatty liver disease, as well as years of research and helping others—whether through coaching or sharing free advice on my blog, Facebook group, and Reddit. This gives me confidence that it's more practical and relatable than much of the other fatty liver reversal content available, especially since some of those books or programs were written by people who haven't dealt with fatty liver directly (either as a patient or as healthcare professionals).

I hope you found it helpful, and I truly hope you'll apply what you've learned to reverse your condition as soon as possible. Be sure to check out my blog, fatty liver reversal page, and the other links below. Don't hesitate to reach out with suggestions or questions—I love receiving feedback, especially the constructive kind (and some praise, too!).

Here are some important links you might want to check

out:

- My fatty liver diary blog/website (where I tracked, followed my progress and wrote hundreds of article about fatty liver disease): https://www.fattyliverdiary.com/

- My Fatty Liver Support group on Facebook (hundreds of people that are/were part of this group managed to reverse their fatty liver disease): https://www.facebook.com/groups/268356693627886

- Discuss Fatty Liver Disease on reddit: https://www.reddit.com/r/FattyLiverNAFLD/

Get healthy and stay healthy!

Made in the USA
Monee, IL
18 September 2025

25961740R00128